Locked-In Synd
Brain Damage

The newest title in the series *Survivor Stories*, this book tells the story of Paul Allen, a photographer who likes opera and was a good baritone singer. At the age of 56 he sustained a stroke that left him paralysed and speechless. He has Locked-In Syndrome (LIS), a rare consequence of brain damage. Although Paul is fully conscious and his cognitive abilities are intact, he is unable to move or speak due to the paralysis of nearly all his voluntary muscles. However, Paul is keen to communicate and through his eye movements he tells his story, from his early life, career, singing and other interests, to the details of his stroke and the effects it has had on his life. The book also includes contributions from Paul's wife Liz, who tells the story from her point of view, along with Paul's physiotherapists, occupational therapists, speech therapists, psychologists and others from the Raphael Hospital who have assisted in Paul's rehabilitation. In telling of his frustrations, his successes, his views on life and how he sees his future, Paul raises awareness of the quality of life possible for those with LIS.

Combining scientific knowledge with personal narrative, this unique and optimistic book is of huge importance to any professional involved in the care of someone with a brain injury, and to the individuals and families touched by LIS.

Barbara A. Wilson is a clinical neuropsychologist who has worked in brain injury rehabilitation for 40 years. She edits the journal *Neuropsychological Rehabilitation*. This is her 27th book.

Paul Allen has lived with Locked-In Syndrome since 2012. Before his stroke he was a singer, photographer, computer programmer and project manager.

Anita Rose is the Consultant Neuropsychologist and Director of Therapies at the Raphael Hospital, UK and also works as an independent consultant across the globe. She has researched and published extensively on brain injury, chronic neurological conditions and multiple sclerosis.

Veronika Kubickova is a trainee clinical psychologist at the University of Oxford, UK. Previously having worked as an assistant psychologist in neuro-rehabilitation, she has helped people re-adjust to life after brain injury. After qualifying, she plans to work with refugee children who have experienced trauma.

After Brain Injury: Survivor Stories
Series Editor: Barbara A. Wilson

This new series of books is aimed at those who have suffered a brain injury, and their families and carers. Each book focuses on a different condition, such as face blindness, amnesia and neglect, or diagnosis, such as encephalitis and Locked-In Syndrome, resulting from brain injury. Readers will learn about life before the brain injury, the early days of diagnosis, the effects of the brain injury, the process of rehabilitation and life now. Alongside this personal perspective, professional commentary is also provided by a specialist in neuropsychological rehabilitation, making the books relevant for professionals working in rehabilitation such as psychologists, speech and language therapists, occupational therapists, social workers and rehabilitation doctors. They will also appeal to clinical psychology trainees and undergraduate and graduate students in neuropsychology, rehabilitation science, and related courses who value the case study approach.

With this series, we also hope to help expand awareness of brain injury and its consequences. The World Health Organisation has recently acknowledged the need to raise the profile of mental health issues (with the WHO Mental Health Action Plan 2013–20) and we believe there needs to be a similar focus on psychological, neurological and behavioural issues caused by brain disorder, and a deeper understanding of the importance of rehabilitation support. Giving a voice to these survivors of brain injury is a step in the right direction.

Published titles:

Life After Brain Injury
Survivors' Stories
Barbara A. Wilson, Jill Winegardner and Fiona Ashworth

Identity Unknown
How Acute Brain Disease Can Destroy Knowledge of Oneself and Others
Barbara A. Wilson, Claire Robertson and Joe Mole

Surviving Brain Damage After Assault
From Vegetative State to Meaningful Life
Barbara A. Wilson, Samira Kashinath Dhamapurkar and Anita Rose

Life After Encephalitis
A Narrative Approach
Ava Easton

A Different Perspective of Life After Brain Injury
A Tilted Point of View
Christopher Yeoh

Locked-In Syndrome After Brain Damage
Living Within My Head
Barbara A. Wilson, Paul Allen, Anita Rose and Veronika Kubickova

For more information about this series, please visit: https://www.routledge.com/After-Brain-Injury-Survivor-Stories/book-series/ABI

Locked-In Syndrome after Brain Damage

Living Within My Head

Barbara A. Wilson, Paul Allen,
Anita Rose and Veronika Kubickova

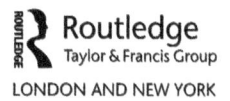

Routledge
Taylor & Francis Group
LONDON AND NEW YORK

First published 2019
by Routledge
2 Park Square, Milton Park, Abingdon, Oxon OX14 4RN

and by Routledge
711 Third Avenue, New York, NY 10017

Routledge is an imprint of the Taylor & Francis Group, an informa business

© 2019 Barbara A. Wilson, Paul Allen, Anita Rose, and Veronika Kubickova

The right of Barbara A. Wilson, Paul Allen, Anita Rose, and Veronika Kubickova to be identified as authors of this work has been asserted by them in accordance with sections 77 and 78 of the Copyright, Designs and Patents Act 1988.

All rights reserved. No part of this book may be reprinted or reproduced or utilised in any form or by any electronic, mechanical, or other means, now known or hereafter invented, including photocopying and recording, or in any information storage or retrieval system, without permission in writing from the publishers.

Trademark notice: Product or corporate names may be trademarks or registered trademarks, and are used only for identification and explanation without intent to infringe.

British Library Cataloguing-in-Publication Data
A catalogue record for this book is available from the British Library

Library of Congress Cataloging-in-Publication Data
Names: Wilson, Barbara A., 1941- author.
Title: Locked-in syndrome after brain damage: living within my head / Barbara A. Wilson, Paul Allen, Anita Rose, Veronika Kubickova.
Description: Milton Park, Abingdon, Oxon; New York, NY: Routledge, 2019. | Series: After brain injury: survivor stories | Includes bibliographical references and index.
Identifiers: LCCN 2018015505 | ISBN 9781138700390 (hbk: alk. paper) | ISBN 9781138700406 (pbk: alk. paper) | ISBN 9781315204727 (ebk)
Subjects: LCSH: Allen, Paul–Health. | Cerebrovascular disease–Biography. | Stroke–Rehabilitation–Personal narratives. | Brain damage–Patients–Rehabilitation–Biography. | Photographers–United States–Biography.
Classification: LCC RC388.5 .W48 2019 | DDC 616.8/10092 [B] –dc23
LC record available at https://lccn.loc.gov/2018015505

ISBN: 978-1-138-70039-0 (hbk)
ISBN: 978-1-138-70040-6 (pbk)
ISBN: 978-1-315-20472-7 (ebk)

Typeset in Times New Roman
by Deanta Global Publishing Services, Chennai, India

Printed and bound in Great Britain by
TJ International Ltd, Padstow, Cornwall

Contents

Preface		ix
Foreword		xi
Acknowledgements		xiii
1	What is Locked-In Syndrome? What causes it? Who is most at risk? Do people recover from this condition?	1
2	Accounts of people with LIS	5
3	Neuropsychological assessments of patients with LIS: How normal is their cognitive functioning?	13
4	Is it always easy to diagnose LIS?	21
5	Paul's journey	28
6	An interview with Liz, Paul's wife	35
7	Treatment at the Raphael Hospital	42
8	Interviews with Paul's friends	58
9	Paul's continuing involvement with music	64
10	Quality of life for people with LIS, and assessing capacity	68

11	Ethical issues in LIS	76
12	Summary and conclusions	81
	References	84
	Appendices	90
	Index	92

Preface

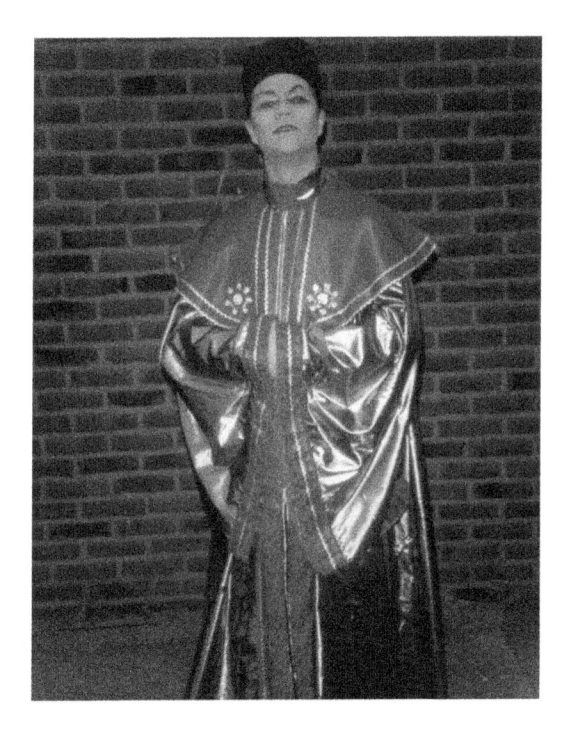

Figure 0.1 Paul in *The Mikado*.

This book tells the story of Paul (Figure 0.1), a photographer and a good baritone singer with a passion for opera. At the age of 56 years, in July 2012, he sustained a basilar artery thrombosis, a stroke in which a clot or blockage develops in the arteries supplying blood to the brain. This left him paralysed and speechless. He has what is known as Locked-In Syndrome (LIS), which means that he is unable to speak and is totally unable to move any part of his body apart from his eyes. All communication has to be made through eye movements. His cognitive abilities, however, are unaffected. He can understand, reason, remember and think.

This is Paul's brief account of himself:

I am a 60-year-old man with Locked-In Syndrome. Before my stroke I was an established wedding photographer with about 200 brides to my name. I set up the wedding photography business in 1996 and traded for 16 years. Although I was principally a wedding photographer, I also offered other types of photography such as child and adult portraits, special occasions, sports events and shows. Of course, I had to limit my commissions as it was my second career. My main job was as a computer project manager. I had eight O Levels and an ONC (Ordinary National Certificate), and an HNC (Higher National Certificate) in Civil Engineering, which is the career I spent the first five years of my working life in. After this I joined the Metropolitan Police Civil Staff as an IT programmer. I also became a cake-maker because somebody told me men can't make cakes!

From the age of 10 until 56, when I had my stroke, I was a singer. My early years were spent singing in my church choir where I became lead chorister. From my 20s onwards I sang with many amateur operatic groups, playing the lead in about 60 operas, operettas and musicals.

My claim to fame was that I sang with the King's College Cambridge Choir in Cambridge Cathedral and several times in the Royal Albert Hall.

Even though it is hard to think of a physical disability more cruel than the inability to speak and to move yet to be fully awake and aware (Laureys 2005), we want to show, through Paul's story, that life is worth living, even after such a devastating event which left him paralysed and speechless. Most able-bodied and healthy people think that they would rather be dead than live with LIS. This is in contrast to what most people with LIS actually feel. Laureys et al. (2005) and others such as Anderson et al. (1993), Doble et al. (2003) and Smith and Delargy (2003) found that people with LIS typically report a meaningful quality of life. Smith and Delargy (2003) state: "The finding that locked-in syndrome survivors who remain severely disabled rarely want to die counters a popular misconception that such patients would have been better off dead" (p. 409). As Beaudoin and De Serres (2010) remind us, people with Locked-In Syndrome are remarkable and a model of inspiration for healthcare teams, as well as for family and friends and others who love them.

Foreword

This is an exceptional book. It tells us the inspiring true story of Paul, suffering from a rare but devastating medical condition called Locked-In Syndrome. A stroke in his brainstem – connecting the brain to the spinal cord – would suddenly, dramatically and forever change his life. From one moment to the other, Paul – a very active and energetic photographer and singer – would find himself fully paralysed and mute. Unable to walk or even move his legs, unable to use his hands or to utter a single word, he suddenly and completely became dependent on others. Needing help to be fed, get dressed, get changed after toilet – he had to accept the help and presence of a carer for all his activities of daily life – 24 hours a day, seven days a week. Especially frustrating was the impossibility to speak, write or express his thoughts and wishes in any way other than through small eye movements. Only his eyes can still be moved by his voluntary control. When asked a question he can communicate "yes" or "no" through an established code. But this means one needs to ask the right and relevant question. Alternatively, when someone spells all the letters of the alphabet he can move an eye and "speak" by selecting letter after letter, word after word. It is a painstakingly slow but important process permitting him to express his own needs and opinions – and even quite often telling jokes. I have never met Paul, but from reading the book I quickly understood he has a strong and rousing personality – at one point in his life he became a cake-maker "because somebody told me men can't make cakes!". In the section written by his friends we can read that Paul "tends to do things with quite a bang". I trust this book will make quite a bang indeed.

Paul's unique story is accompanied by short summaries of other survivors of Locked-In Syndrome, the most famous of whom is Frenchman Jean-Dominique Bauby – author of the international bestseller (and award-winning movie) *The Diving Bell and the Butterfly*. Shortly after the publication of his book Jean-Dominique died from a pulmonary infection (the most frequent cause of death for patients with Locked-In Syndrome). In his living will he had specified that a special association would be created: the

"French Association for Locked-in Syndrome" (www.alis-asso.fr), bringing together many hundreds of patients, which has successfully lobbied for a better care path and reimbursement system and provides practical information and administrative, financial and technical help and assistance for families all over France. I hope that the present book will bring about a similar effect in the United Kingdom and further afield, and will help raise public and medical awareness and optimized protection and care for this rare but devastating condition called "Locked-In Syndrome".

What makes this book so exceptional and unlike the other books by patients with the syndrome is its medical sections and framing, written by psychologist–professor Barbara A. Wilson and colleagues. Barbara is internationally renowned and awarded for her outstanding work in brain injury rehabilitation for over three decades. Officially retired since 2007, she continues to work and inspire the younger generations, doing clinical work, staff training, advising on research projects, acting as editor and publishing prolifically. She actually asked me to write this foreword while she was lecturing in India. Together with Paul, Barbara and her colleagues Anita Rose and Veronika Kubickova offer us a unique opportunity to learn about the clinical challenges of Locked-In Syndrome and related post-comatose states. Alongside the clinical stories of Paul and other patients, we are here offered a scientifically accurate yet readable overview of the current state-of-the art management and care of these vulnerable patients; how to expand the diagnosis and cognitive assessment; improving patient's communication, prognosis, pain and symptom management; and all other rehabilitation challenges, from music therapy over brain–computer interfaces and spasticity to pharmaceutical treatments. This book is a must-read for both the interested lay public and caregivers, including intensive care physicians, neurologists, rehabilitation specialists, biomedical engineers, clinical neuropsychologists, physiotherapists, occupational therapists, speech and language therapists and nurses.

Motor handicap might be maximal in Locked-In Syndrome, yet quality of life can be – and often is – much better than expected and anticipated by many. Paul Allen's inspiring testimony coupled to the medical and psychological expertise of Professor Barbara A. Wilson and her fellow authors will serve to improve the lives of numerous other patients, families and carers in the UK and throughout the world confronted by recovery of consciousness albeit with severe paralysis after coma. *Locked-In Syndrome after Brain Damage: Living Within My Head* is truly an exceptional living testimony of a life worth living after Locked-In Syndrome.

– Professor Steven Laureys, MD, PhD, FNRS Research Director,
Head Coma Science Group, GIGA Consciousness,
University and University Hospital of Liège,
Belgium and Fondazione Europea di Ricerca Biomedica

Acknowledgements

We wish to thank Taylor & Francis for permission to adapt Chapter Two. This chapter is derived from an article published in *Brain Injury* on 1 April 2011, available online: http://wwww.tandfonline.com/http://dx.doi.org/10.3109/02699052.2011.568034.

We also thank the following people: Liz Allen, Paul's wife, for her generous help in preparing this book and for finding the photographs included here; Dr Gerhard Florschutz of the Raphael Hospital for his unwavering support throughout; all the staff at the Raphael Hospital who have worked with Paul, particularly the staff in Tobias House; Paul's friends who agreed to be interviewed; Jessica Fish for her support and help in tracing down references; and Mick Wilson for reading various drafts of the manuscript and for his proofreading.

1 What is Locked-In Syndrome? What causes it? Who is most at risk? Do people recover from this condition?

Locked-In Syndrome (LIS) is a rare consequence of brain damage. Patients are fully conscious but unable to move or speak due to paralysis of nearly all voluntary muscles except the eyes. Communication is with movement of the eyes. Some people can move their eyes up and down (vertically), but not side-to-side (horizontally) (National Organization for Rare Disorders [NORD] 2016). The term "locked-in syndrome" was first used by Plum and Posner (1966). Patients diagnosed with this condition had quadriplegia, lower cranial nerve paralysis, mutism with preservation of consciousness, vertical gaze and upper eyelid movement. According to Bauer et al. (1979), LIS can be subdivided into three types depending on the extent of motor impairment. These are classical LIS, partial LIS and total LIS. Classical LIS is characterised by total immobility except for vertical eye movements or blinking; partial LIS is where some minimal motor activity may be seen, and total LIS is where all mobility is lost, including eye movements, and where consciousness is preserved. Smith and Delargy (2005) point out that because mutism could be interpreted as unwillingness to speak, it was redefined in 1986 as quadriplegia and anarthria with preservation of consciousness.

In 1995, The American Congress of Rehabilitation Medicine noted that LIS had five characteristics, namely (i) sustained eye opening, (ii) preserved basic cognitive abilities, (iii) aphonia or severe hypophonia (loss of voice), (iv) quadriplegia or quadriparesis and (v) vertical or lateral eye movement or blinking of the upper eyelid as the primary means of communication.

LIS is caused by damage to the pons, a part of the brainstem that contains nerve fibres that relay information to other areas of the brain (NORD 2016). Most LIS patients have sustained a stroke in the basilar artery or suffered a pontine haemorrhage (Plum and Posner 1983; Patterson and Grabois 1986). Smart et al. (2008) give six vascular conditions that may give rise to LIS: (i) basis pontis infarct, (ii) pontine haemorrhage, (iii) midbrain infarction, (iv) transient ischaemia, (v) basilar artery occlusion

2 What is Locked-In Syndrome?

and (vi) hypoxic-ischaemic events. They also suggest that there are six non-vascular causes, namely (i) trauma, (ii) central pontine myelinolysis, (iii) tumour, (iv) encephalitis, (v) toxins and (vi) multiple sclerosis affecting the ventral pons. Murphy et al. (1979) also report a case of LIS following a pontine abscess. Nevertheless, according to Schnakers and her colleagues (2008), at least 60 per cent of LIS patients have sustained a basilar artery or pontine haemorrhage.

LIS can affect people of all ages, including children. Males and females appear to be affected in equal numbers (NORD 2016). Beaudoin and De Serres (2010) report that the prevalence rate of LIS is not specifically documented in the literature. They believe, however, that LIS probably represents less than 1 per cent of all strokes. Having said this, they recognise that the incidence rate is probably underestimated. They also believe that the average age of onset of LIS varies between 17 and 52 years old (Doble et al. 2003; Bruno et al. 2008; Beaudoin and De Serres 2010; Casanova et al. 2003). The youngest patients have a better prognosis for survival. In contrast, the website for the National Organisation of Rare Disorders (NORD 2016) state that LIS is seen most often in adults at risk for stroke. This would include people with high blood pressure, those who smoke and those of increased age (Sharma et al. 2016). Because cases of LIS may go unrecognised or misdiagnosed, it is difficult to determine the actual number of individuals who have had the disorder in the general population (NORD 2016).

Although prognosis is generally poor and death can occur through pneumonia or thrombosis, with the right care people with LIS can live for many years, and a few make a good or even a complete recovery. Kate Allatt, for example, was a 40-year-old, very fit, mother of three, who describes her recovery from LIS (Allatt and Stokes 2011). It took Kate eight months to recover from her brain stem stroke. She walked out of hospital by herself to resume her normal life. She still had some difficulties however and continued to improve over the following months. Peter Coghlan, an Australian soldier, was 33 years old when he had his stroke. He documents his recovery over the next six months, when he was able to leave hospital and continue his improvement (Coghlan 2013). Richard Marsh was 60 when he had his stroke and it took him a little over four months to recover to the extent that he could leave hospital (Marsh and Hudson 2014). Partial recovery may also be seen. Kerry Pink, for example, was 35 years old and a mother of two when she became locked-in. After three years she was able to speak again and function, although confined to a wheelchair (Pink 2010). Nick Chisholm, a New Zealand rugby player, sustained his brain injury and LIS on the rugby field. Although he regained a little movement, he remained significantly limited in his independence. Andrew Davies also showed very little recovery. He was only 33 years old when he sustained his stroke.

He spent 10 months in hospital and after three years remained profoundly disabled (Davies et al. 2015). More recovery was shown by Allison O'Reilly (2014). She was 49 years old when she became locked-in. She remained in hospital for a year but when she was discharged home she still required 24-hour care. Three years later, however, she was able to walk and to drive. A rare account of a child who sustained LIS is provided by Pistorius and Davies (2011). Written when he was an adult, Martin Pistorius was 12 years old when he became ill with an unknown illness which left him wheelchair bound and unable to speak. He spent 14 years in institutions. In 2001 he learned to communicate via a computer, make friends and change his life. He continued to make small improvements over many years.

Many people, however, remain with LIS for ever. The best-known case is probably that of Jean-Dominique Bauby, a French man who "wrote" *The Diving Bell and the Butterfly* (Bauby 1997) through painstakingly blinking one eye to his amanuensis. Bauby died just two days after his book was published. An American woman, Julia Tavalaro, published a book called *Look Up for Yes* with Richard Tayson in 1997. Another French man, Philippe Vigand, together with his wife, wrote an account of their experiences (Vigand and Vigand 2000). A British woman, Tracey (Wilson et al. 2011; Wilson and Okines 2014), became locked-in after sustaining a tear in the basilar artery following a fall in the gym when she was 27 years old. She has remained with LIS ever since. We return to these and other accounts in Chapter Two.

To turn to the academic literature, Katz et al. (1992) looked at the long-term survival and prognosis of 29 patients with LIS. They found that survival ranged from just over two years to a little over 18 years with a five-year survival rate of 81 per cent. One study, Casanova et al. (2003), looked at 14 patients with classic or total LIS who were seen three to six months following neuro-rehabilitation. Of the 14 patients, motor recovery was seen in 21 per cent; return of swallowing in 42 per cent; verbal communication in 28 per cent; bladder and bowel control in 35 per cent; and weaning of the ventilator in 50 per cent of the patients. Early recovery from LIS may be seen after recanalisation (unblocking of an obstructed vessel) of the basilar artery (Al-Raweshidy et al. 2011). It may also occur because of fluctuations in the early stages. Hocker et al. (2015) describe a patient of theirs with "a nearly complete locked-in syndrome" (p. 832) whose recovery was monitored. He was weaned off the ventilator and the tracheostomy tube was removed at three months post stroke, by which time he had a severe dysarthria, some head control but no trunk control. At six months, he was able to sit with support of his hands; at 10 months, he was able to ambulate with a walker; at 17 months, he was able to climb stairs. So, although recovery was slow, he was able to achieve a reasonable degree of independence. The same authors say their clinical experience has shown that patients with the classic LIS from pontine infarction may improve, but rarely to functional independence.

In short, recovery does occur for some patients, but for many the LIS is complete and permanent despite some minor improvements. This was the case for Paul, as we shall see later.

2 Accounts of people with LIS[1]

One of the world experts in LIS is Steven Laureys from Belgium. In 2005, he and his colleagues wrote an excellent chapter called "The locked-in syndrome: What is it like to be conscious but paralyzed and voiceless?". The authors state that the earliest report of a patient with LIS in the medical literature comes from Darolles in 1875. Even before that, however, Alexandre Dumas described the condition in *The Count of Monte Cristo* (1844) and Emile Zola described a case in his novel *Thérèse Raquin* (1867). In this chapter we describe accounts of and by people with LIS.

To start with Dumas and *The Count of Monte Cristo* (1844), the character described is a Monsieur Noirtier de Villefort, said to be "a corpse with living eyes". M. Noirtier had been in this state for more than six years, and he could only communicate by blinking his eyes: "His helper pointed at words in a dictionary and the monsignor indicated with his eyes the words he wanted" (Laureys et al. 2005, p. 496). Some years later, Emile Zola wrote in his novel *Thérèse Raquin* (Zola 1867) about a paralysed woman who "was buried alive in a dead body" and "had language only in her eyes". Thus, Dumas and Zola highlighted the locked-in condition before the medical community reported it.

The best-known case of LIS is probably that of Jean-Dominique Bauby, who "wrote" *The Diving Bell and the Butterfly* (Bauby 1997). Bauby had a brain stem stroke in 1995 when he was 43 years old, after which he could only move his left eye. He wrote the book with the help of an amanuensis who used a frequency-ordered alphabet which she recited aloud. Bauby blinked his left eyelid when she reached the correct letter. Unfortunately, Bauby died shortly after the book was published. A highly regarded film has since been made of his story.

Since Bauby's book, there have been a number of others written by survivors of LIS. One of the first to appear after Bauby is *Look Up for Yes* by an American woman, Julia Tavalaro (with co-author R. Tayson). This was also written in 1997. Julia Tavalaro had a haemorrhage in 1966; she was comatose for seven months, during which time she was placed in long-term care. She gradually regained consciousness, but it was not until six years later that her condition was correctly diagnosed. Her mother and sister believed Julia was aware for years before a speech and language therapist, Arlene Kraat, worked out a way of communicating with her. In the book Tavalaro writes movingly of her pain and distress in the years before Arlene Kraat and an occupational therapist began to change her life. She used her eyes to tell of her terrible years "in captivity". Eventually, she was able to use a communication device and wrote poetry. Julia died in 2003 at the age of 68 from aspiration pneumonia.

A French couple, Philippe and Stephane Vignand, published *Only the Eyes Say Yes* in 2000. Philippe Vignand had a stroke at the age of 32 and was in a coma for two months. His wife realised that he was communicating by blinking his eyes in response to her questions, but she had difficulty convincing the staff. One day when the speech therapist was assessing Vigand's gag reflex, Vigand bit her finger, the therapist yelled and Vigand started to grin. Thereupon, the therapist asked "how much is two plus two?". Vigand blinked four times. A letter board was then used initially until Vigand went home and was able to use an infrared camera, which was attached to another camera, allowing more sophisticated communication. The pair discuss Philippe's LIS from their different points of view.

Other books worth mentioning are those by Pistorius and Davies (2011), Allatt and Stokes (2011), Coghlan (2013), Marsh and Hudson (2014), O'Reilly (2014) and Davies et al. (2015). Martin Pistorius (Pistorius and Davies 2011) was a normal, healthy South African boy with a younger brother and sister when he developed an undiagnosed illness at the age of 12. His parents did everything they could to find a diagnosis and a cure, but for many years Martin was "a ghost boy" trapped in a body he could not control, with no voice, no awareness and no memories. He spent his days in a care home but went home each night at his father's insistence. Eventually he woke up; however, he was so severely disabled and mute that nobody realised he was locked-in until one of the staff at the care home came to believe that Martin was aware and insisted he had an assessment to see if he could use an alternative or augmented communication (AAC) system. This began very simply with Martin just looking at pictures, but over several years developed into a sophisticated AAC. Martin never learnt to speak but became proficient with his augmented communication to such an extent that he was able to gain employment and give lectures through a speaking computer. In addition, he gradually learnt some motor control and was able to marry. His story is certainly inspiring.

Kate Allatt (Allatt and Stokes 2011) was a fit mother of three who worked full-time. While out fell running one day she developed a headache, which she ignored. It turned out to be the onset of a brain stem stroke. She tells of the delay in recognising she was conscious and able to understand and think. She also talks of her slow and gradual recovery and the good rehabilitation care she received. Eventually Kate Allatt was able to return home; she was even able to run again. Early on she imagined that one of the nurses had tried to kill her with a "graphite drip" and was told that many LIS patients have delusions early on. This is reminiscent of Tracey (Wilson and Okines 2014), who thought at first that she was in a computer game and had to hide from the nurses. Kate Allatt showed determination and a fighting spirit. These characteristics, however, are only part of reason for her recovery while others such as Andy Davies and Tracey Okines (see below) with the same characteristics did not achieve so much. Nevertheless, Kate's story has been inspirational for many people with LIS, including Coghlan (2013) and Davies et al. (2015).

Peter Coghlan (2013), a British ex-soldier and a bricklayer, developed a brain stem stroke in Australia. Although initially believed to be comatose and unaware, his girlfriend (later to become his wife) said that if he could hear her, he should blink, which he did. So she was the first to believe he was aware of what was happening around him. Coghlan talks about his frustration with the spelling board, which some nurses had not the slightest idea how to use. Tracey (see below) felt the same frustration. It is not difficult for those conversing with LIS people to use a spelling or alphabet board, but it does take time. Coghlan talks about his small early improvements such as his thumb twitching and then learning to swallow. He tells us about the dangers of inhalation pneumonia, which can be caused by too much laughter! Within·two years he was walking and speaking again as well as working full-time.

O'Reilly (2014) is another who made slow improvements over a long time. She talks about brain plasticity, suggesting, for example, that an undamaged part of the brain can take over the function of a damaged part. This is only partly true and of limited value for most adult stroke survivors. Nevertheless, this is another book that is very positive about rehabilitation.

Andy Davies was a successful dentist who sustained his stroke at the age of 33 years. He wrote a book with his wife and mother (Davies et al. 2015). They hoped he would do as well as Kate Allatt but it was not to be. In chapter 14 he says:

> My disability is profound. I have no functional movement in my body below my neck, apart from my right thumb. I can barely speak, and even my eyes do not focus properly. I have no ability to take deep breaths nor clear my throat voluntarily, and my power to select and control an appropriate emotion is almost nonexistent. About the only

two functions that still work properly are my hearing and the reasoning part of my mind.

(Davies et al. 2015, p. 153)

Despite his serious physical disabilities, Andy has a good quality of life. He puts this down to his strong religious beliefs, whereas Kate puts hers down more to "bloody mindedness" and not taking "no" for an answer.

Richard Marsh (Marsh and Hudson 2014), at the age of 60, was a little older than the previous people described above when he had his stroke but, like them, he was in good physical shape; he was a fit man who had been a policeman for many years before becoming a teacher. His description of his paralysis leaving him conscious of what was happening while those around believed him comatose is compelling reading. The life support machines were about to be turned off when he managed to blink and tell those ready to notice that he was cognisant of what was happening. He describes his early care, his fears of drowning in his own saliva and the embarrassment of many of the procedures that had to be performed (such as changing his soiled diaper [nappy]). Unlike many people with LIS though, Richard made a reasonably good recovery.

All these people talk about their fears; their concerns with toileting; problems with feeding, communication and pain; and their difficulty controlling emotions.

In addition to books, there are chapters and papers published. Garrard et al. (2002) describe a woman who developed LIS after a visit to the hairdresser where she had held her head backwards over a sink. She became unwell quickly, but it was five days before the full syndrome appeared.

A rugby player from New Zealand, Nick Chisholm, had an accident on the rugby field; he was taken to hospital and for days nobody could work out what was the matter. Nick wrote: "After six days of going in and out of seizures, after what seemed like all the tests known to man, they said I had had several strokes of the brain stem and then one major one, which left me with the extremely rare condition known as locked-in syndrome" (p. 94). Nick talks about his frustration with the medical staff who misdiagnosed him and gave little hope of improvement. Although he regained a very little movement, he is still significantly limited in his independence despite having his mind and his memory working at 100 per cent (Chisholm and Gillett 2005).

Kerry Pink was a mother of two and only 35 years old when she fell victim to a sudden and unexplained neurological illness which left her paralysed and unable to speak for 18 months. She wrote an account for a newspaper (Pink 2010) in which she said it is hard to explain the torture of LIS. She describes how for months she was on the brink of death, unable to move or communicate. This was followed by three years of moving to various hospitals and institutions. She eventually returned home and although she has to use a wheelchair, she is able to speak.

At the age of 27, Tracey was in the gym showing her daughter how to do cartwheels when she fell and hurt her neck, back and ankle. She suffered from dizzy spells and headaches for the next three days. Her doctor prescribed painkillers for the headache. On the third night she had a seizure lasting more than an hour. Eventually, her boyfriend called an ambulance and she was taken to hospital. A CT scan the following day showed something was wrong deep in Tracey's brain. She was transferred to another hospital for an MRI scan, which showed that she had suffered a basilar artery thrombosis. A neurologist confirmed that the fall in the gym had probably caused a tear in the inner wall of the artery, which in turn caused clotting in the brain. Tracey went back to the original hospital where her parents were told she would probably not survive for more than a few months (Wilson and Okines 2014).

After a month in coma, Tracey began to regain consciousness. About four weeks later a nurse noticed that Tracey's eyes were following her as she moved around the room. Tracey's parents were told that their daughter was aware but her cognitive state was not known. A diagnosis of LIS was made. As Tracey became more alert she was able to answer questions by raising her eyes for "Yes" and lowering them for "No", allowing her parents to communicate with her. Her father accessed the internet and found information from the French Locked-in Syndrome Society. A letter board was described using colours and letters. With some modifications, a similar board was made for Tracey and this is how people communicate with her. The chart is organised with different colours on each row. Each row has certain letters and numbers. Thus, the first row is red and this has the letters A, B, C, D and "end of word"; the second row is yellow and has the letters E, F, G, H and "new word"; the third row is blue with the next set of letters and so forth. The last two rows are white depicting the digits 0–9. First, Tracey is asked to select the colour Red/Yellow/Blue/Green/etc. Once she has raised her eyes to indicate the correct colour, the letters on that line are read to her and thus, the words are spelled out.

This is how Tracey described what happened to her (Wilson et al. 2011):

> *I woke up one morning and my whole life had changed. I get treated like I am stupid. It's patronising. People cannot bother to use the (communication) board as it takes too long. It's frustrating. At the beginning no one knew I could understand and they would talk in front of me. I found out loads of things I shouldn't know. At the beginning I thought I was in a computer game and my aim was to hide from the nurses. Then as I*

> came round from the morphine, reality hit and I realised everything was true. There is no point in me being angry as it won't change anything. I've just got to make the most of a bad situation.
>
> I was told what had happened to me but I didn't take the information in for months as I was doped up on medical drugs. I was on morphine so I was a bit confused with reality and dreams. I remember the room being dark and I could hear sirens outside. People ignored me and talked like I wasn't there. I felt a bit confused as to why it had happened to me. My Dad explained what had happened. Mum and Dad knew from the start that I could understand them. Some of my carers believed this too, but some did not. I felt completely guilty that those who cared for me would have to see me in such a state.
>
> (p. 534)

Although Tracey was able to regain a little head control and a small amount of facial movement, she remains with LIS.

Remember that several days passed between Tracey's original accident in the gym until the full-blown paralysis set in. Several other reports describe cases where patients took several days for them to become locked-in (e.g. Allain et al. 1998; New and Thomas 2005). Allain et al.'s (1998) patient was similar in that she developed a violent headache the day before her husband found her lying unconscious. She became comatose some hours later at the hospital. New and Thomas's patient was admitted to hospital six hours after developing a headache and once in hospital he continued to decline until becoming paralysed and anarthric. Kate Allatt (Allatt and Stokes 2011) had a headache for several days before the LIS developed. Chisholm (Chisholm and Gillett 2005) describes a period of three days between the accident on the rugby pitch and the development of his paralysis. Several of the cases from the Garrard et al. (2002) paper were similar. The woman mentioned earlier who had been to the hairdresser's developed neck pain, nausea, dizziness, clumsiness of the right arm and dysarthria. Five days later a full blown stroke developed. Other cases in the Garrard et al. paper also showed slow onset.

This book tells Paul's story, similar to some of those described above but unique in other ways. Paul's stroke was not so slow as some, as it took place over approximately a 24-hour period.

What happened to Paul?

Paul was born in January 1956. He ran his own business as a wedding photographer (following several other jobs which he mentioned in Chapter One and which are further described in Chapter Five). He was also a passionate baritone singer who was particularly keen on opera. His hospital notes say that in February 2012, at the age of 56, he suffered from a headache which gradually became worse. He felt the pain was located behind his eyes. This resulted in blurred vision, nausea and vomiting. The following day he deteriorated. In the morning Paul had a sudden numbness of his right side running approximately from his earlobe to his toes. He also had difficulty speaking. This episode lasted for about 20 minutes. Paul had a CT scan at the time which found nothing abnormal apart from a "tortuous basilar artery". However, he deteriorated after the scan and had a seizure. Following this he required intubation and ventilation. This means that Paul could not breathe unaided, so a tube was placed into his trachea and connected to a device to enable him to breathe.

The next day Paul was assessed and it was reported in his notes that he was alert and moving his eyes but unable to move any part of his body. He had lost his cough and gag reflexes and his reflexes in general were reduced, especially on the right. A second CT scan showed an occluded basilar artery with low attenuation in the cerebral hemispheres. A tracheostomy was inserted as well as a urinary catheter and a feeding tube. Thus Paul was typical of the majority of patients with LIS in having a basilar artery stroke. His condition, however, was diagnosed very quickly, unlike some of the other LIS survivors we described earlier in this chapter. Paul describes the onset slightly differently. He says that it started with a headache and then two hours later he felt a tingling in two of his limbs. His wife Liz telephoned for an ambulance and he was taken to hospital where he had another stroke that led to the LIS. He thought there were three hours between the two strokes. It was five days before he regained consciousness, but because he had stopped breathing, he was placed in a medically induced coma. Two weeks after he woke up, he was diagnosed with LIS. Paul himself felt that it took Liz one week to realise he could understand. He does not know how she knew this – maybe it was just gut instinct. Over two years later, a medical examination found his physical state to be much the same. It was noted that he had a gross exposure keratopathy of his right eye, which meant he was unable to close it. This had caused some corneal scarring in that eye. There was some concern that this might become infected, causing a corneal abscess and potential loss of this eye. It was suggested that the eye should be taped, especially at night, to help prevent infection. Alternatively, a surgical procedure known as a tarsorrhaphy (a procedure in which the eyelids are partially sewn together to narrow the eyelid opening) could be performed to partially close the eye and give better corneal protection. Paul says he had two eye operations and his bad eye is still getting inflamed. He may have to have that eye stitched shut and, although he cannot see out of that eye, he is scared.

He does not know how long he will have to wait for a decision. Paul's own account of what happened to him can be seen in Chapter Five.

Note

1 This chapter is adapted from *Brain Injury* 2011 (Wilson, B. A., Hinchcliffe, A., Okines, T., Florschutz, G., & Fish, J. [2011]. A case study of Locked-In Syndrome: psychological and personal perspectives. *Brain Injury 25*, 526–538). Permission obtained.

3 Neuropsychological assessments of patients with LIS
How normal is their cognitive functioning?

Preserved cognitive functioning is a prerequisite of the diagnosis of LIS. Although it is true that such patients do not have severe intellectual difficulties, some minor problems are common (Schnakers et al. 2008; Wilson et al. 2011). People with LIS are not easy to assess. They have to blink or raise their eyes to communicate, so tests are required where patients can indicate "Yes" or "No" (typically eyes up for "Yes" and down for "No" or blinking once or twice for "Yes" and "No"), and/or can spell out answers through a communication board. Spelling out in this way is slow and so is not suitable for all tests; prose recall, for example, would take too long, and, of course, motor tests and tests of speed are not appropriate.

Some studies use communication devices controlled by eye movements (e.g. Allain et al. 1998), although most use eye movements for Yes/No plus a communication board. Patients may tire easily with eye movements (Smith and Delargy 2005) and there may be additional visual or hearing problems (Trojano et al. 2010; Smart et al. 2008; Smith and Delargy 2005). Despite these limitations, neuropsychological testing has been carried out with LIS patients. In most studies, relatively few tests have been used and the results are mixed. The first reports of neuropsychological assessments of LIS patients would appear to have been those of an Italian patient (Cappa and Vignolo 1982; Cappa et al. 1985). They found that their patient, who had been in the locked-in state for 12 years, had normal intelligence. A similar finding was confirmed in two cases from France, a man and a woman, reported by Allain et al. (1998).

The first study to suggest that there might be some minor cognitive deficits was from Schnakers et al. (2004) in Belgium. They tested five patients who had been in the LIS for between three and six years and 10 control participants. Interestingly, the control participants had to respond with eye movements. All were assessed with modified versions of digit span to assess working memory. The Doors and People Test was used to assess episodic memory; and the Wisconsin Card Sorting Test to measure executive functioning.

A test of phonological and lexico-semantic processing, a vocabulary test, and tests to measure sustained and selective attention for auditory stimuli were also given. Although for most measures the patients' performance was in the normal range, differences between participants were found, as well as some deficits. Schnakers et al. (2004) state that "LIS patients recover a globally intact cognitive potential" (p. 314), but may remain with some cognitive deficits.

Smith and Delargy (2005) carried out a review of the literature on the LIS and found that attention, executive function, intellectual ability, perception, and visual and verbal memory can all be affected. In one study of 44 patients with LIS, eight reported memory problems and six showed difficulties with attention. Memory impairments were reported as being more likely when the aetiology was traumatic (Leon-Carrion et al. 2002). Garrard et al. (2002) assessed seven patients with isolated brain stem lesions. Although they had sustained damage to the pons, they did not have LIS. Up to seven cognitive functions were assessed (frontal/executive; attention; general intellectual ability; naming; visual memory; verbal memory and perception). The number of cognitive domains affected ranged from one to six; thus all seven patients were shown to have deficits in at least one cognitive domain. Another paper from the Belgian group (Schnakers et al. 2008) assessing 10 LIS patients found that none had deficits in tests of verbal intelligence but impairments in one or several tests were found in five patients, three of whom had additional cortical or thalamic lesions. Signs of fatigue were seen in two patients.

A study by New and Thomas (2005) reported three neuropsychological assessments carried out at six, 12 and 24 months following a basilar artery occlusion in a man who was in his early 30s. Although the man *had* been locked-in, he was not in this state at the time of the assessment. Indeed, he was discharged home at seven months post stroke and at that time was walking with a stick. Unusually for LIS patients, he went on to make a good recovery. Nevertheless, this study is rare in reporting follow-up assessments. The authors note a number of cognitive deficits including reduced speed of information processing, perceptual organisation, executive skills and attention. This patient, however, was unlike others described here as he was not paralysed and could manipulate material.

The presence of cognitive deficits in patients with LIS was confirmed by Rousseaux et al. 2009. They gave 19 tests to nine LIS patients and two groups of control participants; seven with frontal or fronto-temporal lesions and 16 neurologically intact people. Significant differences were found between the LIS patients and the healthy controls on auditory recognition, oral comprehension of complex sentences, delayed visuo-spatial memory, mental calculation and problem solving. The authors conclude that although

LIS patients are by and large cognitively intact, some cognitive deficits are to be found.

Smith and Delargy (2005) report that hearing is usually well preserved in these patients, although visual difficulties such as blurring and diplopia may be present. However, in 2008, Smart et al. reported a man with LIS together with cortical deafness. He was assessed using written instructions. His performance was in the normal range for most tests but he was impaired on the California Verbal Learning Test. A LIS patient with unilateral spatial neglect has also been reported by Trojano et al. (2010). This patient underwent scanning training and was then able to use a communication device.

The conclusion from these studies then is that there are no severe cognitive deficits in patients with LIS, but some cognitive functions are outside the normal range.

The most detailed neuropsychological assessment (prior to Paul's assessment) would appear to be that of Tracey (Wilson et al. 2011). Tracey is described in Chapter Two. She was seen two or three times a month for several months. Communication was through eye movements. Tracey was either asked questions to which she responded "Yes" or "No" or else she spelled out words using her communication letter board. Although Tracey is quick, this method is still much slower than normal speech so certain tests were inappropriate. Each session lasted for about one hour. Sometimes Tracey was seen alone and sometimes two of us (the neuropsychologist and the speech and language therapist) saw Tracey together, with one presenting the test material or questions and one writing down the letters and checking with Tracey that we had recorded accurately what she wanted to say. Smith and Delargy (2005) remind us that patients initially tire quickly when using vertical eye movement to communicate and in the first few weeks or months their attention span may be severely limited. Tracey was two years post stroke when the neuropsychological tests began and she concentrated well.

The cognitive assessment addressed (1) premorbid functioning, (2) language and naming, (3) memory, (4) visuo-perceptual functioning and organisation, (5) visuo-spatial functioning, (6) executive functioning and (7) non-verbal reasoning.

The report on her neuropsychological functioning concluded that Tracey was of at least average ability prior to the incident and that she was still functioning well in most areas. Indeed, her executive functioning as measured by the Modified Card Sorting Test (Nelson 1976) and the Brixton Spatial Anticipation Test (Shallice and Burgess 1997) was exceptionally good. On tests of naming and language as well as basic visual perception and visual spatial processing she showed normal functioning. There were two areas where she appeared to have some difficulty: the first was in some aspects of visual memory and the second was with some more complex visual perception organisation and reasoning tasks.

These deficits were seen in tasks involving visual processing, organisation and reasoning tasks. Her basic vision was obviously unimpaired as she was able to do the visuo-perceptual tasks on the VOSP with little difficulty. When the material became more complex however, as with Picture Completion and the Manikin test (a test of visual mental rotation: Ratcliff 1979) she scored well below average or in the impaired range.

Other LIS patients have also been reported as having problems with perception (Smith and Delargy 2005; New and Thomas 2005; Garrard et al. 2002). In addition, Smith and Delargy (2005) remind us that visual problems are not uncommon. Tracey appeared to have diplopia and blurring of vision and this could have added to her problems in processing complex visual material. One apparent discrepancy is with the two matrix reasoning tasks. On the Matrix Reasoning from the Wechsler Adult Intelligence Scale-IV (Wechsler 2008), Tracey scored in the average range, whereas on the Ravens Matrices (Raven 1982) she scored below average. These tasks seem similar in many ways and both involve visual reasoning. One difference is the Matrix reasoning is smaller with less scanning involved. It is also in colour and it is possible the stimuli are more discriminable and less subject to the effects of diplopia or blurring of vision.

Another area of difficulty for Tracey was visual memory. Her scores on both the recognition memory for faces (from Warrington's Recognition Memory Test 1984) and recognition of doors (from Baddeley et al.'s Doors and People Test 1994) were poor. Although she scored normally on the picture and face recognition subtests from The Rivermead Behavioural Memory Test-3 (Wilson et al. 2008), these are simpler stimuli and less demanding tests than the first two. So once again, it is with complex visual material that Tracey has problems. Again, visual memory difficulties have been mentioned in other studies (e.g. Smith and Delargy 2005), so Tracey was not unusual.

Her memory for verbal material that was read to her was very good. She remembered all the words on the California Verbal Learning Test (Delis et al. 1987) by the fourth trial and retained them after a delay. Indeed, when seen the following week, Tracey spelt out that she could still remember all the words. The normal presentation of this test is for the participant to say back all the words he or she can remember and Tracey had to spell them out. We thought at first this might disadvantage her, as the later words could "fly away" while she was spelling the first ones, but in retrospect the spelling out may have helped her to process them at greater depth. Even so, she had good recall on Trial 1 where she had to retain the words in memory before spelling them out. What is clear is that she scored exceptionally well and had no obvious memory difficulties. Her autobiographical memory as measured by the Autobiographical Memory Interview (Kopelman et al. 1990) was also normal. One verbal memory task where she scored below average was the recognition memory for words subtest from Warrington's (1984) test, but this was also a test where she had to read the words so may have been affected by the visual processing difficulty described above. Tracey rarely forgot where she was up to when spelling out sentences with the communication chart, unlike those interacting with her (we had to write down each letter to prevent confusion and loss of memory for what had gone before). Tracey seemed to have a particularly strong working memory.

On the two tests of executive functioning administered, Tracey scored very well, making only two errors on the Wisconsin Card Sorting Test and scoring in the superior range on the Brixton Spatial Anticipation Test where she has to discover a rule to predict the location of a coloured circle. Although this is a visual test, the stimuli are clear and easy to discriminate.

The cognitive assessment then is consistent with other reports of people with LIS, although in some ways, Tracey appeared to have a higher level of functioning than many. She was also assessed in more detail.

In addition to the cognitive tests, Tracey was assessed with the Hospital Anxiety and Depression Scale (HADS; Zigmond and Snaith 1983) to measure her emotional well-being; the Short-Form-36 Health Survey (Ware et al. 2000) was administered to assess her quality of life (QOL) and the Visual analogue scale (VAS; Huskisson 1974) was used to measure her perception of pain.

On the HADS, Tracey scored only 1 for the depression items and 5 for the anxiety items. Neither of these scores are abnormal; there is no suggestion that she is depressed or particularly anxious. Tracey, herself, agreed with this when the scores were fed back to her. On the VAS for pain rating, she said she could feel pain normally anywhere in her body; she rated her headaches as 85 on a 0–100 scale and said she had this pain about four times a week. The pain was described as "heavy and severe". She believed her headaches were caused by her posture and a visiting pain expert said she thought this explanation was probably correct. Tracey's head was supported in a headrest, but due to her decreased head control and her strong cough reflex, when she coughed her head fell forward, causing increasing strain on the neck muscles. Following the pain assessment, Tracey had rest breaks during the day and this reduced the severity and frequency of her headaches.

On the SF-36 measure, Tracey's scores were obviously low because she was unable to do anything for herself. Nevertheless, she felt her general health was much better now than a year earlier (it was over two years since she developed the LIS) and she had far fewer respiratory infections since admissions to the rehabilitation centre. She did not rate herself as having any emotional problems and believed she had a reasonable QOL. Emotionally, then, it would seem that Tracey was a well-balanced young woman with no obvious depression, anxiety or other mood issues despite the severe limitations placed on her because of her almost total paralysis. She became frustrated at times because some people were unwilling to use the communication method. This was understandable. She also said that she felt afraid and insecure at times because she could not see around her but her main message was that there was no point being angry and she just had to get on with life.

As we wished to replicate Tracey's assessment, Paul was assessed with many of the same tests as Tracey. His eyesight, however, was much worse so some tests could not be administered. These included the matrix reasoning and the picture completion subtests from the WAIS-IV and the object decision subtest from the VOSP. Poor eyesight may have been responsible for poor scores on other subtests too. The results can be seen in Table 3.1.

In many ways, Tracey and Paul score similarly: both scored in the above average range on a test estimating premorbid functioning, both have good language skills and both are above average on tests of executive functioning. Neither has severe memory problems, although they have some mild difficulties with recognition memory (Tracey with faces from the RBMT and Paul with doors from the Doors and People test. Their basic visual perceptual skills are adequate, although both struggled with some aspects of visual reasoning and visual problem-solving tests (picture completion and Raven's Matrices). This is probably because of eyesight problems: Tracey has diplopia and blurred vision while Paul has poor acuity. The main difference in cognitive performance was on the Manikin Test, a test of mental rotation. Tracey struggled with this whereas Paul had little difficulty, making only two errors from a maximum score of 32.

In short, these assessments confirm earlier studies that people with LIS have no severe cognitive deficits although some minor problems may sometimes be seen. This may be due to sensory problems such as poor eyesight or to other brain lesions.

Schnakers et al. (2008) believe that "additional brain injuries are most likely responsible for associated cognitive deficits in the LIS" (p. 233). Tracey's scan showed some cortical atrophy and Paul's scan showed an occluded basilar artery with low attenuation in the cerebellar hemispheres. Low attenuation is a spot that appears on a radiographic image as less dense than the surrounding healthy tissue. The significance of this is unclear.

Table 3.1 Summary of neuropsychological test results

Test	Tracey	Paul
Estimate of premorbid functioning		
Spot-the-word (from the Speed and Capacity of language processing; Baddeley et al. 1993)	Above average	Above average
Language and Naming		
Test of Reception of Grammar-2 (Bishop 2003)	Normal score	Normal score
Graded Naming Test (McKenna and Warrington 1983)	Average	Above average
Memory		
Recognition Memory Test (Warrington 1984)		
Words:	Low average	Low average
Faces:	Impaired	Average
Doors recognition memory subtest (Baddeley et al. 1993)	Borderline	Impaired
Picture and face recognition subtests from The Rivermead Behavioural Memory Test-3 (Wilson et al. 2008)		
Picture recognition:	Good average	Good average
Face recognition:	Average	Borderline
California Verbal Learning Test (Delis et al. 1987) Maximum score on any one trial = 16		
Total recall	Above average	Average
Delayed free recall	Above average	Average
Categories	Above average	Average
Autobiographical Memory Interview (Kopelman et al. 1990)		
Personal semantic	Normal scores	Normal scores
Autobiographical incidents	Normal scores	Normal scores

(*continued*)

Table 3.1 Continued

Test	Tracey	Paul
Visuo-perceptual functioning and organisation		
(From Visual Object and Space perception Battery: Warrington and James 1991)		
Screening test	Pass	Pass
Incomplete letters	Pass	Pass
Silhouettes	Pass	Pass
Object decision	Bare pass	Abandoned (poor vision)
(From Wechsler Adult Intelligence Scale-3: Wechsler 2008)		
Picture Completion	Below average	Abandoned (poor vision)
Visuo-spatial functioning		
(From Visual Object and Space perception Battery: Warrington and James 1991)		
Dot counting	Pass	Pass
Position Discrimination	Pass	Fail (poor vision)
Number Location	Pass	Fail (poor vision)
Cube Analysis	Pass	Pass
Manikin Test (Ratcliff 1979)	Impaired	Unimpaired
Executive functioning		
Modified Card Sorting Test (Nelson 1976)	Above average	Above average
Brixton Spatial Anticipation Test (Shallice and Burgess 1997)	Superior range	Very superior range
Non-verbal reasoning		
Matrix Reasoning (from the Wechsler Adult Intelligence Scale-3: Wechsler 2008)	Good average	Abandoned
Ravens Standard Progressive Matrices (Raven 1982)	Below average	Below average

4 Is it always easy to diagnose LIS?

With people like Paul, Tracey and the others described in Chapter Two, it is easy to diagnose LIS because they all communicate with their eyes. This makes it relatively straightforward to establish a Yes/No response and, as we saw in Chapter Three, there are many neuropsychological tests which can be administered. Earlier, in Chapter One, we learnt of the five characteristics of LIS spelt out by The American Congress of Rehabilitation Medicine which are, to recapitulate, (i) sustained eye opening, (ii) preserved basic cognitive abilities, (iii) aphonia or severe hypophonia (loss of voice), (iv) quadriplegia or quadriparesis and (v) a vertical or lateral eye movement or blinking of the upper eyelid as the primary means of communication. However, there are occasions when it is not entirely clear whether or not a patient has LIS. This may happen, for example, when eye movements are compromised, making it difficult for certain patients to communicate effectively with their eyes. Other patients, despite having a lesion in the pons, (like all LIS patients), may *also* have some cortical damage, leading to their cognitive abilities being compromised. Just as it is easy to misdiagnose the vegetative and minimally conscious states, with some 40 per cent of patients diagnosed as in coma when they are not (Annen et al. 2017), it is also difficult to determine whether a patient has or does not have LIS. Leon-Carrion et al. (2002) pointed out that it takes, in most cases, up to three months to diagnose LIS after a stroke or brain injury. It can, of course, take much longer, sometimes even years for a correct diagnosis to be made – as we saw with Julia Tavalaro and others in Chapter Two.

We discuss here two patients with whom we remain uncertain as to whether to diagnose LIS. Their two cases are presented in some detail to illustrate the dilemmas clinical neuropsychologists may have when trying to diagnose this condition.

The case of M.A.

The first patient is a 39-year-old man, M.A., who developed a sudden headache while driving home from work. He collapsed, was taken to hospital and, following a CT scan, was diagnosed with a pontine haemorrhage. Thus his lesion was indicative of a diagnosis of LIS and many of the staff thought this was accurate. A neuropsychological assessment, however, suggested this could not be reliably determined. We first saw M.A. 10 months post insult, when he was unable to move his limbs and his left eye was closed for most of the time. He appeared to see out of his right eye and was able to blink with it. So far, so good – all these behaviours were consistent with LIS. His mother tongue was not English, so for part of his assessment M.A. was seen in physiotherapy by a physiotherapist who was able to speak to the man in his native language.

We assessed M.A. with the Wessex Head Injury Matrix (WHIM), a behavioural observation tool consisting of 62 items in a roughly hierarchical order from least to most difficult, which provides a sequential framework of behaviour covering a patient's level of responsiveness and interaction with the environment. Behaviours observed and noted by the WHIM may occur either spontaneously or in response to sensory stimulation. The WHIM can monitor small changes from coma through to emergence from post-traumatic amnesia in patients with traumatic brain injury (TBI; Shiel et al. 2000). Marjerus et al. (2000) also report its use with stroke patients. On the WHIM, M.A's highest ranked behaviour was 14 (mechanical vocalisation – where any sound such as a yawn or sigh scores a point) out of 62 possible behaviours. This score was considered to be an underestimate of his true ability as there were many things he was unable to do because of his paralysis. Additionally, it was hard to interpret his blinking, which, we were told by other staff, was his means of communication.

In order to determine whether or not M.A. had a reliable Yes/No response, we asked him a series of simple questions requiring "Yes" or "No" answers (for example "Is your name Jonathan?" and "Are you a man?"). Although we were told that he blinked twice for "Yes", people differed regarding their assessment of his "No" response. Some of the staff said he blinked once for "No" while others said he did nothing for "No". On our questions, he *appeared* to blink two or three times to some questions, but he also blinked two or three times when *no* questions were asked. The blinks were not strong and seemed to be more like a fluttering of the eyelid. Our conclusions were that there was no doubt that M.A. was awake and, at least to some extent, aware. Nevertheless, despite the fact that many people, including a medical doctor, were convinced he had LIS and the fact that he *sometimes* blinked twice when asked some questions, this response was not always consistent. The blinks were very rapid and easy to miss. Some people, when asking questions, made an opening and closing movement with their fingers to indicate blinking, so it is possible that M.A was imitating the gesture rather than answering the questions. Other people with LIS show a much

Is it always easy to diagnose LIS? 23

clearer blink, rather than a rapid fluttering of the eyes, making it easier to be sure that they are responding to the question asked. We were not implying that M.A *did not* have LIS, simply that the evidence was not clear cut. Reports from staff working closely with the patient reported that he was more responsive when his wife was present. At that time, we had not been able to observe him with his wife. Consequently, we felt it was difficult to be absolutely sure that this man had LIS and we needed further evidence to obtain certainty.

We arranged to see the man's wife and other members of the family when they were interacting with M.A. to see if more consistent Yes/No responses could be obtained. Unfortunately, there was no change in M.A's behaviour. M.A. was seen again a few weeks later, with his main carer present. She had established a good relationship with him. Interpreting the blinking remained of concern to us, and although we would have preferred eyes up for "Yes" and down for "No", blinking had been established and was therefore accepted. The trouble was his "blinks" were more a quivering of his eye rather than a clear-cut shutting. At times he seemed to really answer "Yes" but he also frequently blinked several times for this response, not just twice and, on occasion, he blinked several times for "No" too. Furthermore, he sometimes blinked several times when he had not been asked *any* questions. His carer felt he had problems controlling his eye muscles so could not make a clear-cut single response. This view coincided with our own, which was that any evidence remained unclear. We continued to be bothered by our inability to come to a conclusion and although many of the staff were sure M.A. had LIS, as neuropsychologists, we felt we required firmer proof.

Two months later, a visiting doctor, experienced in assessing patients with LIS, was asked to examine M.A. Like us, the visitor was of the opinion that he had some awareness. His right eye looked towards the person speaking, though he could, of course, have been responding to voice rather than because he understood the command "Look at…". It was confirmed that his eye movements were hard to interpret and the following suggestions were made:

1. Use an eye patch to control for the double vision. We tried this but it did not help us to determine Yes/No responses more reliably. Furthermore, it was not clear that M.A had double vision.
2. Use cards with a tick for "Yes" and a cross for "No" to see if that helped clarify his ability to answer Yes/No questions accurately. This did not help either.
3. The bobbing of the eyes exhibited by the man might be helped by Gabapentin or Pregabalin (if these have not yet been tried). He had already been tried with this and it did not help. Botox was discussed

but, as this was not considered to be functionally helpful, the idea was abandoned.

A few weeks later, M.A was seen for the final time before his discharge to a long-term care facility. He was able to open his left eye to a greater extent than previously. However, he still seemed to have better sight in his right eye and this was the one he used to make eye contact. He appeared to be trying to talk and made a fair amount of noise orally. This time, instead of trying to use blinking to communicate, we used Yes/No cards as suggested by his speech and language therapist (we held one of the cards above the other). This seemed to help a little and we felt this made his responses easier to interpret. Nevertheless, his eye movements were random and we found ourselves giving him the benefit of the doubt on more than one occasion.

His highest ranked score on the WHIM was now 28 (looks at object when requested). On the Yes/No questions (from the 9 questions suggested on his communication chart), he scored 7/9 correct (although on some occasions he was given the benefit of the doubt because it was not entirely clear if he was looking at the correct card; this was because his good eye tended to wander around). Nevertheless, he was certainly above chance. We still felt we could not be sure that he had LIS and that he was communicating reliably. In a research institute or teaching hospital, one might have been able to use more sophisticated equipment such as an EEG (which is normal after LIS), but this man was seen in a rehabilitation hospital with limited access to such facilities. In retrospect, he had undoubtedly emerged from the minimally conscious state but almost certainly had cognitive problems, plus brain stem damage and ophthalmoplegia (poor control of his eye muscles). Even the medical doctor who had first thought M.A. had LIS now changed his mind, saying he did not have LIS.

The case of U.P.

The second patient, U.P., was also a puzzle, although we felt we had a slightly better understanding of him. This man was of a similar age to the previous one, being 40 years old when first seen. Once again the neuropsychological assessment began when U.P. was 10 months post insult. He had been involved in a motorcycle accident resulting in a subarachnoid haemorrhage, a prepontine bleed, a skull base fracture, plus numerous other fractures. As well as a tracheostomy, a ventriculoperitoneal (VP) shunt was inserted after U.P. developed hydrocephalus.

During the assessment, U.P. was always awake and appeared to be alert. He had some rhythmic mouth movements but did not verbalise. His left eye was partially stitched closed because he was unable to blink that eye.

His right eye stared intently at people. Because he had nystagmus, it was not always easy to know if he really was looking at something or not. On occasion, he was given the "benefit of the doubt". This time, it was not the other staff insisting he had LIS but our own suspicion that he might have this. Our conclusions to the first assessment were that he was definitely awake and alert, was responsive to sound and appeared to look at objects when requested. Even though we believed he might have LIS, it was impossible to establish a Yes/No response in order to confirm this. We tried getting him to blink for "Yes", then asked him to raise his eyes for "Yes" and finally asked him to look at "Yes" and "No" cards (first when these were side by side and then when they were placed one above the other in case of scanning difficulties). With each attempt, U.P. just looked at the tester. On the basis of the results at that time, we suggested he was at the top of the minimally responsive range – or that he had just emerged from this state. Because we were not 100 per cent sure our scores were reliable (that is to say we did not know if he was really looking from one object to another or whether it his nystagmus making his eyes jump), we said we would repeat this assessment in a few weeks' time. The repeated assessment showed no changes in his behaviour. It was still not clear if he was really looking at a named object or whether his nystagmus made it appear as if he were looking. U.P. did not try to communicate; and a Yes/No response could not be established. Once again it was concluded that he was functioning at the top of the minimally responsive range.

At all times, however, we were worried that we were underestimating U.P.'s level of functioning. His good eye stared so intently at one, and he was always so alert, that we questioned our diagnosis. Then his wife discovered he could read! Of course, someone who can read is well beyond the minimally conscious state. U.P was much better at the written word than the spoken word. As this is unusual in patients with naming and language disorders (which we thought U.P. might have), it raised questions about his hearing. In retrospect, his ability to hear should have been one of the first things to check for, but clinical experience suggests that relatively few people are deafened after a brain injury while many have problems with visual acuity and visual perception. U.P. had an audiology examination and the report said that he had bilateral severe to profound sensori-neural hearing loss, worse on the left side; he also had a glue ear on the left. Once communication was established, via the written word, U.P. himself denied having problems with his hearing. It is unclear why the audiology report said he had a hearing loss while U.P. himself felt he did not.

It is possible that another reason he was better at the written than the spoken word was because of delayed processing or because of ataxia or some other reason. Once it was realised that U.P. could read, he was provided with an iPad on which questions were typed for him in large letters. When next assessed by us, his iPad was used. We began by explaining the purpose of the assessment to him. This was written out in simple language. The questions we wanted to ask were then typed out one at a time. At first, he was asked to blink again, but he did not respond. Yes/No cards were used to no effect. Discussions with his speech and language therapist followed and we were told he could not blink but he could raise his right eyebrow very slightly for "Yes" and could indicate "No" by an almost imperceptible shake of his head. Because the movements were so slight, we needed three sessions observing him making his Yes/No responses to ensure we could interpret these behaviours correctly. Finally, we were able to assess him with the Putney Auditory Comprehension Screening Test (PACST: Beaumont et al. 2002). He passed four of the five practice items and all of the biographical items but made some errors on the other questions (for example he responded incorrectly to the questions "Is cyanide poisonous" and "Was Picasso a train driver?"). Although U.P's score of 49/60 was well above chance, he certainly had some cognitive problems. This was confirmed by another assessment, Cognitive Assessment by Visual Election (CAVE; Murphy, in press). The CAVE assesses people who have emerged from a disorder of consciousness but are too impaired for traditional tests. There are six categories (objects, numbers, words, letters, pictures and colours). In each category 20 stimuli are presented, two at a time and the person being tested is asked to look at (or indicate), the correct one of each pair. Thus, a ball and a bus may be presented and the person asked to look at the "BUS". Half the stimuli are on the right and half on the left. U.P scored 7/10 on objects; 7/10 on numbers; 8/10 on words, 10/10 on letters; 10/10 on pictures and 10/10 on colours. In each case the instruction was written out on his iPad (for example, "Please look at BUS"). Additional cognitive deficits are, perhaps, unsurprising as he had several skull fractures sustained in the road traffic accident as well as his pre-pontine bleed. Thus, as well as pontine damage, U.P. had cortical damage too. So, in this case, it would appear that U.P. had at least partial LIS plus additional cognitive problems.

In conclusion

Both M.A. and U.P. would appear to have ophthalmoplegia, making it difficult for them to control their eye muscles. This, in turn, of course, means that it is hard to establish communication. As we saw in Chapter One, there is a condition called "Total locked-in syndrome, or completely locked-in state" (Bauer et al. 1979). This is a version of LIS where the patient's eyes are paralysed in addition to the limbs and body. Neither M.A. nor U.P. had paralysis of the eyes; they were both able to open their right eye with the left partially opened in M.A.'s case and more or less fully closed in U.P.'s case. A neurologist might have been able to say more about the eyes; as Pierrot-Deseilligny et al. (2004) report, a neuroscientist can tell much about the organisation of the brain through eye gaze abnormalities. They also remind us that eye movements are controlled by ocular motor nuclei in the brain stem. In a clinical situation though, without recourse to sophisticated equipment, finding the best way (or indeed any way) to converse is problematic.

One of the American Congress of Rehabilitation Medicine's criteria for LIS is communication by eye movement. While it can be argued that M.A. tried to do this, his ophthalmoplegia prevented him doing this adequately. U.P., on the other hand, was unable to do this. He could just about raise his right eyebrow for "Yes", but could not voluntarily control his blinking or raise his eyes up or down. Does this mean that M.A and U.P did not have LIS? We cannot be sure with M.A but we are of the opinion that with U.P. that he may, indeed, have partial LIS but also have additional cognitive problems. The American Congress of Rehabilitation Medicine states that basic cognitive abilities are intact with LIS patients, but this begs the question, what are basic cognitive abilities? Is it the ability to understand? Does it include memory, naming and attentional problems and so forth? We have already seen in Chapter Three that people with LIS have *some*, albeit mild, cognitive difficulties. Duffy (2000) says that in LIS the individual is conscious and sufficiently intact cognitively to be able to communicate with eye movements. So he seems to be implying that the ability to communicate is sufficient with regard to cognition. U.P. can communicate, if not by eye movements then by marginal movements of his head. The point we want to make here is that it is not always easy to determine LIS, and we feel it is possible for some patients to have LIS plus other cognitive problems.

5   Paul's journey

Like most people I was very young as a baby, so I don't remember anything. What I do remember is my mother telling me that when I was a few months old my sister dropped me on my head, which probably explains a great deal. Ironically, prior to my stroke I have only been admitted to hospital twice in my life – the first time was when I was three years old. I was taken to hospital to have a circumcision, which was needed for medical reasons. The morning after the operation I woke up in a general ward and shouted at the top of my voice, "My willy hurts!" The nurses were not very pleased.

I grew up in a council-owned prefab in South Norwood with my parents, my sister and two brothers. We had no central heating, so in the winters I was bathed in a tin bath in front of the fire. I still can't believe my father took a photograph of it! I had a very close relationship with my mother, although I imagine I caused her a lot of headaches as a child by constantly arguing with my younger brother, Nigel. This was not so much the case with my father, however; we rarely saw eye to eye. Despite this, I do recall some funny stories, which still make me smile. One of my favourites is of the time when Dad invited our neighbour and his son to our house for Guy Fawkes Night, which we celebrated with a fireworks display. Dad was not ready to be outdone by our neighbours' vast selection of fireworks, so he saved a very impressive-looking rocket for last. He fitted it in a milk bottle, which turned out to be a grave mistake. In the crucial moment, the bottle toppled over and the rocket shot across the grass, through the fence and landed in our next door neighbours' runner beans. Our neighbour, "Old Beans", watched his pride and joy rise up in flames and turn to ash. I'm sure Dad must have been mortified, but I could not stop laughing.

Sadly, my father passed away at only 65. My mum then decided to move down to Devon, where she spent some of the happiest years of her life, and I have many fond memories of visiting her frequently. Over time Mum developed a great sense of humour and we were often in stitches together. I recall one time when I was painting Mum's new house in Devon; I was so busy talking to her whilst on the stepladder that I didn't realise the pot of paint had caught on the guttering. As I was coming down it tipped over and poured all over my head. I shut my eyes quickly and continued to stand glued to the ladder with paint dripping down my face for a good while. It was only when Mum was done laughing that she went to look for a towel.

I was also very close to my brother Dave, who was 10 years older than me. Despite this age difference, we got on very well – I guess he was my hero. I suppose that I was destined to become a biker from the age of seven, when I used to ride to school on the back of Dave's racing bike. It felt good to see some of my friends standing at the school gate waiting for my arrival. This early exposure to biking only grew as I became older; I bought my first bike at the age of 17 and I rode for 29 years. During this time, I owned 12 bikes, ranging from a 90cc Suzuki Trials bike to a 1200cc Yamaha Sports Tourer. I used the bigger bikes to tour central Europe extensively and I made separate trips to the Isle of Man, Scotland, Wales, Ireland and the West Country. I also visited Dave in Holland on my Yamaha before my wedding and asked him to be my best man. My brother Dave was taken from us in a tragic car accident at only 38 – before my wedding took place – leaving our family devastated. He was also in a choir, not the same one as me; he took it more seriously. He had a group in Holland called the Dave Allen band.

I am reasonably close to my younger brother Nigel, but not as much as I was to Dave. He does have his funny moments though, and there is one in particular which still gets me laughing now. When we were living in South Norwood our next-door neighbour had an enormous German Shepherd dog called Caleb. At that time, Dad used to be very skinny, to the point of his ribs showing. One scorching day, Dad was sunbathing in the garden. When Nigel saw him, he shouted, "quick Mum, call Dad in, Caleb might think he's a bone!" In that very moment Caleb jumped over the fence – I've never seen Dad sprint that fast in his life. He ran into the shed to hide.

I was always fond of my sister Janet, but never more so than now, which is ironic because she currently lives in France. When she still lived in Little Chalfont near Amersham I used to love visiting her and her husband Phil, and my nephews Tim and Nick. I often played games with the boys and I recall one time when Tim and I were competing at a game of snooker in the loft, which was recently boarded and carpeted. Phil failed to mention that not all parts of the floor were boarded, so when I stepped back to take my winning shot, my leg went right through the bedroom ceiling. What a sight it must have been from down below!

I loved my nan and granddad. Granddad used to wear a pair of hearing aids which he would conveniently turn off when Nan was nagging him. I was only ten when Granddad died and I remember hiding behind the settee so no one would see me crying.

30   Paul's journey

To say that my professional life has been varied is probably an understatement, for I have been a paperboy, a milkman's assistant, a housing engineer, a structural engineer, a computer programmer, a systems analyst, a photographer, an actor and a singer. My qualifications are reasonable; I got eight O-levels and after leaving school I joined the Greater London Council (GLC) to train as a civil engineer. Through GLC's sponsorship I attended college one day per week, eventually obtaining an Ordinary National Certificate (ONC) and later receiving my Higher National Certificate (HNC) from the Polytechnic of South Bank. During my first year I worked in a housing engineer's office and my main job was working on an architect's drawing of an estate in Thetford. In my second and third years I worked in the structural engineer's and city district surveyor's offices. I was eventually asked which office I preferred, and relocated to the district surveyor's office in Shoreditch. I started completing my HNC endorsements in order to make it equivalent to a university degree. What I didn't realise at the time was that the institute of civil engineers had changed their membership policy and therefore only accepted applications from degree candidates. Having chased this dream for several years, their decision left me disheartened and annoyed. I soon changed my employers as well as my career and joined the civil service as a trainee computer programmer. After several months of arduous interviews and exams I joined the Metropolitan Police Service (MPS) as a computer programmer and worked for them for 21 years. This might seem like a long while to work for one company but in that time I was a systems analyst, a computer installation planner, a purchaser and a project manager. During one of my jobs with the MPS I enjoyed setting up the computer room, but I soon found the day-to-day running tedious. I eventually escaped and joined the Installation Planning Team. Our main responsibility was the planning of major installations and purchases of equipment or systems. Having taken a course in Systems Analysis was infinitely helpful! I got promoted to the police project manager and joined the Crime Report Information Service to work on an Inner London Magistrate Court Service project. The project involved the installation of a computer at each court using a specialised system, which allowed the courts to communicate with their associated police stations. A few years later I went on to design a system which further simplified the inputting of a charge or summons on a computer and additionally allowed the user to access editing facilities. With all that training under my belt, in 1996 I started a business called Paul Allen's Wedding Photography! It all began as a favour for my girlfriend's best friend. Although she had a professional photographer booked for her wedding, he did not have a back-up. A week before the wedding I received a panicked phone call, asking if I could take over as the photographer had broken his arm playing football. I borrowed a good camera, familiarised myself with the controls and before I knew it, I was photographing the entire wedding. I was pleased with the results and I think other guests must have been too as I began receiving phone calls asking if I could photograph their weddings. I traded for 16 years, alongside my everyday job as a computer project manager, photographing nearly 200 weddings. Although I was principally a wedding photographer, I did offer other services such as adult and child portraiture, show photography and product shoots. I also photographed a cleaning firm, but it was difficult to make a feather duster look interesting. At the age of 44, whilst still working for MPS, I was out-sourced to a large American company. My claim to fame with them was to act as project manager for the prison service, the department of work and pensions and the British Petroleum account. With the 2008 recession well underway and inevitably, the company being taken over by a larger company, I was offered voluntary redundancy. So, at the age of 53, I accepted early retirement, which gave me more time to expand my wedding photography business and to pursue my singing and acting. What a shame it is that I only had three years before my stroke. Over the years, I have photographed weddings at some fairly prestigious places, including Buxton Palace, Eltham Palace, Lincolns Inn – where many of the high court barristers have their chambers – and Wellington Barracks, which is opposite Buckingham Palace and home to the Royal Scots Guards.

Music has always been an inseparable part of my life. Already at the age of four I was using a tennis racket as a guitar to entertain relatives with Lonnie Donegan songs. At the age of 10 I joined a church choir (I stayed for 25 years) and I was soon singing most of the solos – someone had to! Some years later, a very persuasive lady called Veronica convinced me to sing a duet with her in a competitive festival and to my great surprise we won the gold medal. Encouraged by this early success, I decided to enter several solo classes. A couple of years later Iona, my singing teacher, formed a group made up of four singers and I was delighted to be asked to be the baritone. Over a period of about ten years we performed many charity concerts but the one of which I am most proud raised £3,500 for charity. Some of my fondest memories are of singing in the Rock Choir at the Royal Albert Hall, singing with the choir of King's College, Cambridge and at my friend's wedding in Cambridge Cathedral. I was a boy soprano when my voice broke; I had to stop for about a year, then rejoined the choir as a bass.

Coupled with a passion for singing, acting has formed a significant part of my life. At 12 I was cast as Oliver in a school production. It gave me my first taste of the stage and has stayed with me throughout my life. I have performed in about 60 shows which include opera, operetta, musicals and plays with incidental music. Most of the shows are amateur but some were pro-amateur. It is difficult to select my favourite three shows, but if forced to I would choose **Sweeney Todd, Pirates of Penzance** and **Chicago**. *Chicago was a very lavish production with a strong cast and performed at the Churchill*

Theatre in Bromley. I played the part of Amos Hart or "Mister Cellophane", a part which taught me the potential power of pathos. It is possible to portray a pathetic character in such a way that the audience are all on your side and are compelled to feel sorry for you. The Churchill boasted a 54-foot-wide stage, making it one of the widest non-opera house stages in Europe. It was used by travelling theatre companies and by companies wishing to try out their production prior to moving to the West End. I have played the Pirate King in Pirates of Penzance *a few times* (Figure 5.1), *but my favourite production was with Medway Opera Company*. They were a big talented company who used a very large theatre in Chatham. It was also my first professional part, so it means a lot to me. Probably my most favourite show of them all was Sweeney Todd, *which I performed at the Bob Hope Theatre. When Bob Hope was alive he was the chief patron and benefactor of the theatre, so the company consequently changed the theatre's name to his.*

The Bob Hope theatre was not particularly large, offering only 200 seats, but it is intimate and wonderful to perform in. The show had an extremely

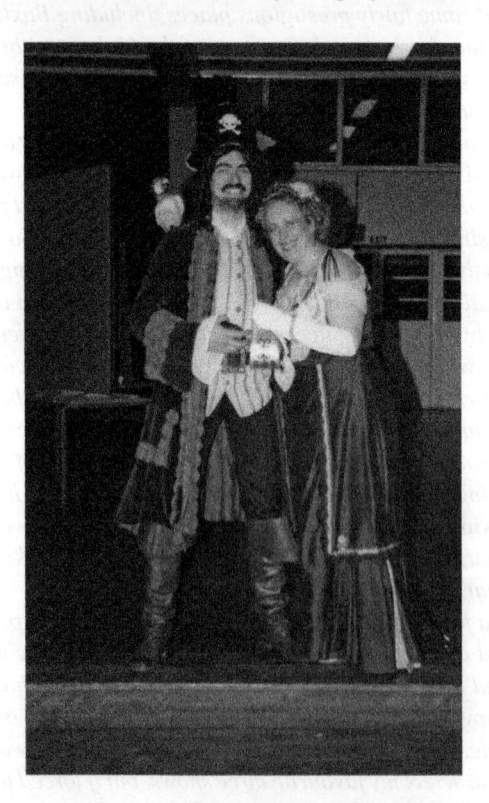

Figure 5.1 Paul in *The Pirates of Penzance*.

strong cast, which made me very proud to be playing the leading role. It ran for two weeks and sadly my mother died in the middle of the run. She was only 70 and I was devastated to receive the news. It made the second week very difficult but the cast were very supportive. I was playing the most demanding part of my life at a very traumatic time but with encouragement from the cast, especially my leading lady, the show was very good.

I have been married twice. It is not something of which I am proud, but it just happened. My first marriage ended when I was 37 and I met Liz (Figure 5.2) in 2000 whilst performing in The Beggar's Opera. The following year I took Liz to Rome. I had bought her an enormous engagement ring, which I kept hidden for three months before I proposed. I sat her down on the edge of the Trevi Fountain in the sunshine and proposed to her in Italian. I still wonder whether she understood a word of what I said! We were married at our local church in Eden Park in 2002. The wedding day was idyllic; the weather was fine and the day was filled with music and great friends for company. Iona, my singing teacher, put together a quartet to sing for us during the signing of the register, and even my former choir master came out of retirement to play the organ for us. During the dinner, we were serenaded by an all-female string quartet and in the evening, we had a live band. One of our friends generously offered a villa in Ibiza for our honeymoon; it was splendid. Liz and I shared some lovely holidays since, Goa and Tenerife to name a few. We will both be old, but I secretly hope Liz and I can make it to our Golden Wedding anniversary.

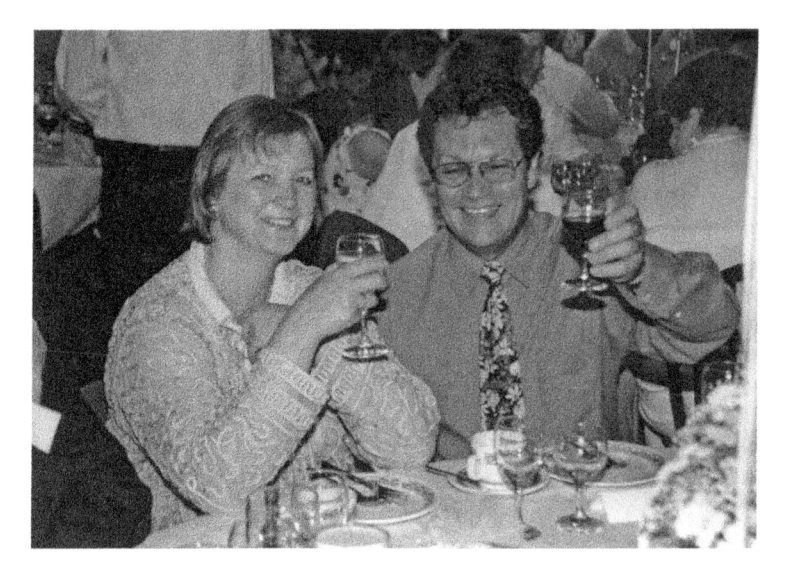

Figure 5.2 Paul and Liz.

No one expects to have a stroke and I was no exception. Yet on 3 July 2012, that is exactly what happened to me. In the early hours of the morning I awoke with a tingling sensation all down one side and a headache on the other. I must have dozed off because when I woke up again, the pain and tingling reversed to the other side. Liz was very concerned so she phoned for an ambulance. By the time the paramedics had arrived, I had started vomiting, so they rushed me into hospital. Once I arrived I was assessed and sent for a CT scan. After the scan, I was waiting in a corridor for a porter to take me back when I had a massive stroke. A nurse found me and took me to a doctor in the Accident and Emergency department (A & E) where I had yet another stroke. I stopped breathing. Luckily, A & E were quick to act; they resuscitated me, attached me to a ventilator and put me in a medically induced coma. I woke up five days later in the Intensive Care Unit (ICU). I spent seven weeks in ICU, paralysed and unable to speak. During this time I was told that what I was suffering from what is called "Locked-In Syndrome". They also said that no National Health Service (NHS) hospital could provide the rehabilitation that I needed.

Fortunately, Liz found the Raphael Hospital near Tonbridge, Kent. It is a private hospital which accepts NHS-funded patients. I was admitted to Tobias House, which specialises in high-dependency patients. The staff are looking after me very well and the grounds are superb. They are well kept and even have a lake.

I miss all my past life; I would be a fool to say otherwise. However, there is a positive aspect to my stroke; it has given me plenty of time to examine myself and decide how I could improve. It has also reminded me how much I love my wife. I have been blessed with many good friends; to date, I have had 120 visitors at the hospital and 20 who visit me at home during weekend stays.

Apparently, there are fewer than 400 people with Locked-In Syndrome in the UK. With those sorts of odds I could have won the lottery.

Of all the things that have helped me in my hour of need, the most significant are:

> My faith
> My wife
> The staff at Raphael
> My friends
> And my sense of humour.

I hope I recover because there are many people and places I want to see and things to do. Besides, it has been years since I last had a beer.

6 An interview with Liz, Paul's wife

Liz (Figure 6.1) was asked, "Can you tell me about the lead up to Paul's stroke?"

She replied: *We were having some work done at home, as usual; it was a conservatory. We had a lovely Victorian House which we had spent loads on, time and money but we loved it. The people next door were having some work done on their roof and some pitch fell on the new glass roof and Paul got very stressed about it. Paul did suffer with stress and depression as well. On the Monday morning he woke up and said he had a dreadful headache, so he stayed around at home and didn't do very much.*

On Tuesday morning Paul woke up and said, "I still have a headache but it has changed, I am all numb down one side." To me that was an alarm bell, so I said I was going to phone for an ambulance. "Don't be so stupid," he said, "it is the wrong side for a stroke." I said, "It doesn't really matter what side it is, I am phoning for an ambulance," which I did, and it came and they were very good. They said, "Have you any pets? If so shut them up." But I didn't have time: as I put the phone down there was a ring on the door bell and they were there, so I had to hurriedly shut the dog up, who was very friendly. So then they came in. Paul was walking and talking at this point, but he then started vomiting, quite a lot. They said they didn't think it was a stroke because he passed all the tests – you know, the arms up, the smile and he knew where he was and everything and he walked onto the ambulance. On the ambulance he said that after a while the numbness came back – I wasn't with him as I followed in the car – and he started to feel peculiar, so he said to the people, "I can't talk now, I just feel odd." He went into the hospital. I had to find a parking space as you do, and I got into the triage bit where he was and there was a lovely nurse who sent him for a CT scan. I had to then go and move the car, as you only get a couple of hours, and I found another parking space which was okay but I didn't have a lot of cash to put into the machine so I went back to the triage. The nurse

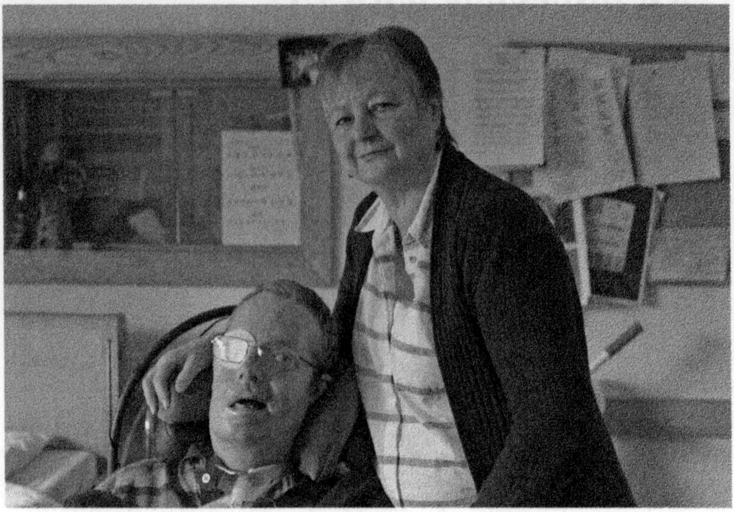

An interview with Liz, Paul's wife

Figure 6.1 Paul and Liz in 2018.

came to me and said, "You know, he has been gone an awfully long while. I will go and see what has happened." She was gone for a while and then she came back and said, "I don't want to worry you but he has deteriorated, so I have taken him nearer the doctors," as he was in a corridor outside the CT scanner room in the x-ray area waiting for a porter to bring him back. He had obviously had a stroke then. She took me to where he was so that I could see him. He was all bent and twisted and he couldn't vocalise. He was making sounds trying to speak but he couldn't he was all sort of shhhhhhh, sssssss, and he couldn't get words out. I had to go and put money in the car meter again. When I came back he had obviously had another stroke because they were rushing him into resus (resuscitation) because he had stopped breathing and stopped everything. So I followed, streaming in tears and everything; it wasn't very nice. They put him onto life support and put the tube down to breathe for him as I think he had stopped and they put me into a side room so I could sit and sob, which was nice of them. When they were ready they came to tell me they didn't know what it was because he had the CT scan before he had the stroke. They took him up to intensive care and I followed. He was on everything, you know bits all over him, the machines were beeping. There was no point in me staying there; I stayed as long as I could but he was in an induced coma, so I went home in the evening. People were coming in saying "have a gin and tonic or something", and I thought I could do but I didn't know if I would get a call. So I went in the next day

An interview with Liz, Paul's wife 37

and he was still in the coma, wired up. After a couple of days they woke him up and he really wasn't himself. He couldn't speak, he couldn't move, he couldn't do anything. This day they sent him for another CT scan, he didn't have a MRI because they said he couldn't with all the wires on him and he needed those and so they then saw the stroke. It was in his brain stem and there was a clot underneath. I found a letter this year from the hospital saying that by the time they found it, it was too late to give him the clot busting drug which would have helped him. Up to that point they told me it could be encephalitis or something else. But then they saw the stroke and told me that is what is was. Then his sister came over with reams of paper as she thought it might be Locked-In Syndrome and she spoke to the doctors who said, "Yes it is." She then got depressed and I had to take on the strength to keep going. It wasn't easy because to start with Paul wouldn't respond, he didn't want to know.

The next question to Liz was, "Do you think he didn't want to know or was it at that stage he couldn't respond?" She said: *He could respond. I know that because he really upset me because he wouldn't respond, and I cried with one of the nurses and he heard me and from that moment on he started to respond. He started to do things I was asking him to do.*

"What kind of things?" Liz was asked. She replied: *The speech therapist had given me some things to do with Paul – a finger of a rubber glove with ice to stroke his face to try and make him open his mouth and to move his tongue. From then on he did start to do this."* We said, "How long after the stroke was this?" to which Liz responded, *"This was about a week, maybe two weeks. Then I had an awful episode with the doctor as I had to apply for power of attorney (POA) as it was a second marriage for both of us and we both had our own little accounts which we hadn't merged, and Paul had all the monies to finish of the conservatory in his account and I didn't have enough to do it in my account so I applied for POA. This awful doctor – he wasn't Paul's consultant but he was one of the consultants on the stroke unit – he came up and was very rude. He stood on one side of the bed and totally ignored me and started talking to another doctor with him, saying they have applied for POA, and so I interrupted and said "I am Paul's wife" and he said "Yes I know" and came round to my side of the bed and said, "You have applied for POA." I said, "Yes, there are things I have to do at home and I need to do it." He said, "Aren't you working, can't you pay for it?" And then looked down at Paul and in a very harsh tone of voice said, "Do you know what happened to you, do you know where you are, do you know what hospital you are in?" Paul did the only thing he could do: he shut down. So the doctor turned round and told me "He is on his way out now" and I thought, what? He took me into a side room and said,*

An interview with Liz, Paul's wife

"Paul is dying and how do you feel about that." What did he expect me to feel about that? Was I expected to jump up and down? I was really upset and there was a poor little nurse with me, she hadn't met me, she hadn't met Paul before that day as she had come in from another hospital as they were short staffed, and she was really upset at his treatment. The doctor continued saying, "Well he has had pneumonia," and I thought what – has he really got pneumonia? This was the first I heard of it. I knew he had had chest infections but he [the doctor] continued saying, "He has pneumonia and he isn't going to last much longer," and then he left. He left leaving me in pieces and the other doctor said, "When we say pneumonia we do mean chest infection" – in a manner of trying to help – and this poor nurse asked if I was okay. I said no, but then said, "Let me wash my face and I will come back in." I was really, really upset. Another nurse who knew Paul and knew me made me a cup of tea and said, "Don't worry we all know Paul is responding," and she apologised and the sister came to apologise and the next day four others came to apologise. When Paul left I did write to the rude doctor telling him never to speak to anyone like that again. I didn't put in a complaint, I had no idea what his medical skills were, but his bedside manner was atrocious. This was about three weeks after Paul had the stroke.

Next, Liz was asked, "How did you know Paul could respond?" She told us: *He could blink, blinking for yes and no and the speech therapist was showing me how to use this ice exercise but there wasn't always ice so we couldn't always do it. So I tried and that is when I introduced the whisky to him just on a swab and it did make him move his tongue because I put it round his lips and he had to find it. It was pleasurable to Paul, so it provoked a response.*

"How long was he in hospital for?" we asked Liz. *He was in Bromley – the Princess Royal Hospital (PRUH). He was there seven weeks, he was getting sort of physio every other day for about half an hour – passive movement. But every time I visited I would rotate his feet, move his legs up and down, I did what I could as I had a background as a physio assistant, so I knew he needed to keep moving so I did what I could. One of the funny things was I brought an electric toothbrush (a battery one) to use on his feet, in between his toes around his toes – using it to stimulate to try and get some movement, and when I came here (the Raphael Hospital) I realised that they were using it on his teeth! He did have a little bit of movement, I would rotate his hands and move his arms. Then we had the battle of where he was going to be transferred to. They said (the doctors and the speech therapist), "He has to go to Putney, it is the only place that will help him. He has got to go there." So I drove over there with my sister-in-law one Sunday morning. It took me over two hours to get there and that was on a Sunday. I wasn't impressed; they wouldn't let* us look at anything, we could only walk down a corridor and have a cup of tea and look at the gardens. I came home and my sister-in-law went home by public transport, which took her over two and a half hours, so I thought, this was no good. I then came to the Raphael to have a look.

Liz was then asked, "How did you hear about the Raphael?" She answered: *"They were the two places that were offered but they were pushing Putney – I didn't have a say in it, I didn't know anything about anything. They said Putney was the best and he had to go there, but I decided to make an appointment to see the Raphael and I was shown around and it was really good and I thought this is a really nice place, the way they deal with the patients and visitors. It was really nice and I thought, I wouldn't mind him coming here, but they were very anti it at the PRUH; but then he was discharged to the Raphael. I thought it strange they were pushing Putney but then he came here (the Raphael). This was seven weeks after the stroke and I am glad he came here, it is a much better place. He came on 20 August. He had the stroke on 3 July 2012.*

The next question to Liz was, "When he first came here what was different?" Liz replied, *He got more therapy and people were talking to me. The staff were talking to me; the physio staff talked to me, which was important because Paul didn't see the point in doing anything – for example, what was the point going on the tilt table – so I had to explain to him why. We both have a faith, which is very important to us, and I feel that whilst I was not happy with the physio I used to work with when I was a physio assistant, I believe I was sent there because this was going to come up in our life and I would need the understanding and knowledge. So I was able to explain to Paul it was going to help and then he did it! Everything that happened, staff spoke to me, they told me what was happening – you never got to see any of the staff apart from nursing staff at PRUH. Everyone here was very friendly and very helpful. When Paul was admitted here I got here before him and I was met by Sister Mary, who was gorgeous. I was very emotional and she just made me a cup of tea and talked to me like a normal person. This just helped; she didn't say anything profound, she just chatted. Gerhard comes and chats to you, everyone is very open and friendly, which is nice. Gerhard knows all the families and patients, which is good – you wouldn't get that in any hospital.*

The following question to Liz was, "When Paul came here did he start using a communication aid?" *Yes*, she said, *it was the OT here who introduced it. They had tried to use one in Bromley but it was too difficult, but the OT here looked at it and with Paul was able to simplify it, divided the alphabet into three so Paul could blink at the right place, it was so much easier. At the PRUH they used a coloured board and certain letters were allocated to certain colours, but for Paul it was not helpful and was not easy. He tried* but he couldn't use it. To start with he didn't have a tracheostomy. At PRUH he was incubated and then they told him he had to have one, which he was worried about as he wanted to sing again, but they said, "It is fine, it won't interfere with your vocal cords and when it comes out you will be fine and you will only have a little scar," so he was okay about that. After it was fitted he looked like he had been attacked by Sweeney Todd, because he was on aspirin, his blood was thin and blood just poured out of his neck. Initially he didn't want to see people, but I made him see people and I stayed and helped with communication, which was fine.

"How did you meet Paul?" Liz was asked. *I lived in Pakistan with my first husband for around five years, as he was a customs officer and was involved in stopping heroin getting out of the country. While we were out there we separated but we had the children (boy and girl) and so I came home in 1993 as a single parent and had to find somewhere to live and a job, which I did. Then, because I needed something to do, I joined a drama group, which was great as I could take the kids there. Initially I thought I would make the costumes, but I found myself on stage and that went on for some time. In 2000 they were doing* The Beggar's Opera *and I thought I would not audition, I would do backstage and front of house. Paul was invited in because he has a brilliant voice, baritone, to sing the part of Mr Peacham. My friends knew me as a quiet person and a good listener and they knew Paul could speak for England so they decided to get us together and see what would happen. It was an instant thing when we met, and we found our paths had been crossing throughout our lives. We were born in the same hospital; Paul's birthday is five days after mine but he is three years younger. I used to run for Croydon and he and his mates used to hang around where I was training and we both sang in the Croydon School's Choir at the same time and we rehearsed at his school but he would have been 12 at the time and I would have been 15, so I wouldn't have noticed him. Later on, after I came home from Pakistan I worked at a school in Deptford and after I left the school I worked in a care home. Paul did a concert at that school to raise funds for the school, but that was after I left. Then* The Beggar's Opera *happened and Paul and I met. We got married in 2002. He proposed by the Trevi Fountain in Rome, Italy. We met on 21 June 2000 and he proposed April the following year. We married in July 2002. The children then were 18 and 19. One was at university and one about to go.*

We asked Liz how her children responded when Paul had the stroke and were told, *They wanted to rush down and see him but Tracey lives in Middlesborough; she wanted to come down straight away but had to go back the following day, so I said no, and Robert as well was phoning, wanted to come, but I said no. They phoned every day, however, to make sure I was okay and Paul was okay, and they came the weekend after the stroke. I kept everyone away until I knew what was happening. They have a good relationship with Paul. Initially, when we first met they were younger teenagers and it wasn't all that brilliant but now they have a good relationship. Paul would have loved children but we share a grandson and a granddaughter now.*

The penultimate question to Liz was about their friends. We said, "Paul and you have very good friends – have they remained consistent throughout?" Liz replied, *Most of them have remained, a few have dropped away. They have known him longer than I have, they have been singing with him for years and there are lots of people who are very close to him and I have tried to include them in everything that goes on, so I joined Facebook to make sure that everyone can follow Paul. They were devastated when Paul had his stroke. His singing teacher, Iona, is a lovely lady, she is 82 now and she was heartbroken. She comes to see him all the time. She was going round all the churches she could find saying prayers. At one point there were 15 churches that had Paul on their prayer list. His friends have organised concerts, including one to develop his garden so when he goes home he can access his garden and enjoy it.*

The final question asked Liz to say more about her faith. She said, *Without my faith these last four and a half years would have been awful, but when I drive home from visiting Paul I have a quiet word with God; it is my faith and I don't expect others to have it, but it is important to me. When Paul gets home on a Sunday we go to church because the people at church enjoy seeing him. There is a group from church who come down to see him when they can. Faith for me and Paul is very important. Paul started singing at the age of 10 in the church choir, which is where he got the bug for singing from. He sang all through his teenage years into his 20s and early 30s in the church choir. Paul is one of those people, if he is in the room of 100 people and 99 say Paul that was really good with one saying "I think you could have done that a bit better", he will listen to that one. His self-confidence is not all that good. I suspect that comes from his parents. I never met them as they died before I met Paul, but listening to Paul, he didn't get on with his father although to be fair, his father didn't get on with any of his children. When Paul went out to work he was invited to leave home. He was told to get his own place and pay for himself. This happened with no explanation, so that is what he did. He used to go home for Sunday lunch but his father would ask him what he was doing there. So I think his lack of self-confidence comes from the relationship he had with his father. He has a good relationship with his siblings who visit. He had an older brother who died.* Paul provides some of this information in Chapter Five.

7 Treatment at the Raphael Hospital

The Raphael Hospital is a unique, independent hospital, specialising in the neuro-rehabilitation of adults. The philosophy, based on Rudolf Steiner principles, follows an approach which believes in the integration of mind, body and spirit. It is used in a number of fields, including agriculture, teaching, arts and medicine. In rehabilitation, it is used to support people suffering from complex neurological disabilities, including physical, cognitive and behavioural impairment. Otherwise known as anthroposophic medicine, it complements and is integrated with mainstream medicine (Wilson et al. 2016).

Paul was admitted to the Raphael Hospital in August 2012 and remains an inpatient at the time of writing (January 2018). Throughout his stay, and to this day, and in addition to medical and nursing care, he receives physiotherapy, speech and language therapy, occupational therapy, neuropsychology, external applications including rhythmical massage and embrocations, art therapy and music therapy. Early on, a system was devised to enable Paul to communicate. The letters of the alphabet are in sets, so set 1 includes the letters A–H, set 2 includes I–Q and set 3 the remaining letters (set 4 is numbers). To communicate with Paul, one says "Set 1?", "Set 2?", "Set 3?". Paul blinks his left eye for "Yes". If he has chosen "Set 1", the communicator says "A?", "B?", etc. Words are spelled out in this way. Paul does try to mouth words, but it is not clear to many people what he is trying to say. Some people, especially his wife Liz, are good at interpreting his mouthing, but the spelling of letters is safer, by and large. Once the communication system was established, it was made clear to staff that Paul has full mental capacity and is able to communicate all his needs using his communication system. He is involved in his daily routines and can decide what he wants to do.

We summarise the involvement of these different disciplines.

Medical report

Although it has already been described as to what happened to Paul (Figure 7.1), the medical report is included here to give the medical doctor's point of view.

Mr Allen was well until 02/07/12 when he started with a headache. The headache was gradually worsening, located behind his eyes and associated with blurred vision, nausea and vomiting. He had no neck stiffness or rash. The headache continued to worsen until his admission to the accident and emergency (A&E) department at his local hospital. On the morning of 03/07/12 he suddenly experienced numbness down his right-hand side from earlobe to toes, which lasted approximately 20 minutes. His wife reported he had some speech disturbance transiently as well. By the time the local ambulance had arrived the symptoms had resolved. He had a further episode of numbness in the ambulance.

On arrival in Accident and Emergency his Glasgow Coma Scale score was 15/15, with no focal neurology; however, on the basis of the history he had a CT (computerised tomography) scan. The scan was reported as NAD (nothing abnormal discovered) but with an addendum of a tortuous basilar artery. Following his scan he acutely deteriorated and had what appeared to be a tonic-clonic seizure. He desaturated, was intubated and brought to the intensive treatment unit (ITU) for ventilation.

On ITU a lumbar puncture was performed, which came back as NAD except for a slightly raised protein. Overnight he was kept sedated and ventilated. The following morning the team attempted to wake him with a view to extubate as his examination and bloods were pristine. Unfortunately, he did not seem to be able to move, although he was alert and moving his eyes. His cough reflex, which had been previously present,

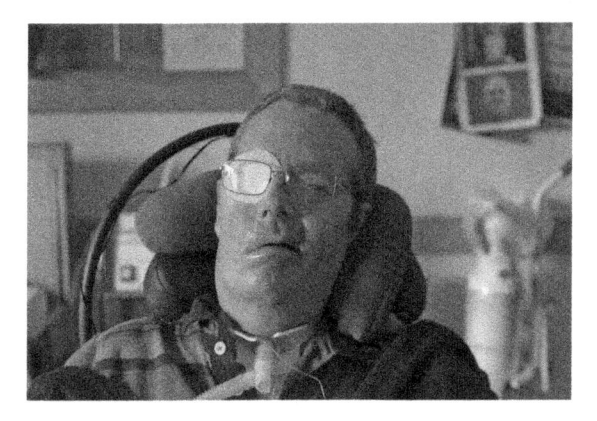

Figure 7.1 Paul as he is today.

was lost. His neurology at this time was of widespread flaccid paralysis, reduced reflexes (especially on the right), equivocal plantars and no gag reflex. A second CT angiogram was completed after consultation with the neurologists, which showed an occluded basilar artery as far as its termination, with otherwise unremarkable vasculature. There was also low attenuation in the cerebellar hemispheres. A diagnosis of Locked-In Syndrome was made.

He was reviewed by the neurologists and stroke consultants; in discussion with King's neurosurgeons and stroke team. Sadly, it was felt that it was too late for thrombolysis or any other intervention. A tracheostomy was performed on 07/07/12 and a percutaneous endoscopic gastrostomy (PEG) was inserted on 13/07/12. He is currently on NIPPY-3 (a type of ventilator). Since then he continues to be entirely ventilator dependent and not able to take his own breaths.

An examination of the central nervous system (CNS) functions showed there was no meningism or nystagmus, although there was a right ptosis (drooping of the eyelid). When PERLA (pupils equal and reactive to light) was assessed it was found that the left pupil was slightly more dilated than the right (cranial nerve 2). A corneal reflex was present (cranial nerve 5). There was a partial palsy of the third and sixth cranial nerves. The fourth and seventh cranial nerves were difficult to assess but appeared to be intact. His swallowing (cranial nerves 9 and 10) could not be assessed but seemed to be impaired. Other cranial nerves were very difficult to assess in detail, but seemed to be intact. He had quadriplegic flaccid paralysis. The deep tendon reflexes for both upper and lower limbs were very brisk. Sensation was again difficult to assess in detail, but seemed to be intact. There was no clonus and no fasciculation (muscular contractions and spasms), nor was there a Babinski sign.

Nursing report

The following recommendations were made from the nurses.

Nursing recommendations

Paul to continue Nippy assessment from Breas Medical (*This is a ventilator*).
Plans to make regarding Routine Tracheostomy tube changes every 4 weeks.
Urine dipstick to be done once in a week or as necessary.
Blood test to be done according to GP recommendations.
Paul should be weighed weekly or at least fortnightly.
He requires good suction machine, pulse oximeter, suction catheters, tracheostomy dressings and holders, cuff manometer and tubings to go with the Nippy machine.

Regular positioning when in bed.
Full assistance with ADLs.
PEG feeding and management.

Current medication

- Adcal-D3 efferv Tabs – one daily
- Citalopram Oral drops 40 Mg/Ml – five drops daily
- Clopidrogrel 75 Mg tabs – one tab daily
- Movicol 13.8 G Sachets – one on alternate days
- Selsun shampoo – Twice a week

PRN medication

- Dyoralite sachets
- Maxitrol eye drops
- Maxitrol eye ointment
- Hyaback ocular lubricant 0.15%
- Hydrocortisone 0.1%
- Metaline dressing 8cm × 9cm
- Metoclopramide 5Mg/ 5Ml oral soln
- Paracetamol 500 Mg Tabs
- Saline Nebuliser liquid 0.9% 2.5ml
- Salbutamol Nebuliser liquid
- Capsaicin 0.025% cream
- Cardioron 5% Ampoules
- Cavilon Durable barrier
- Co-codamol 30/500 Tabs
- Diazepam rectal solution
- Fleet Enema
- Trimovate cream

Nutritional status

Paul is seen regularly by dietician for his feeding regime.

Paul has 4 × 125ml 2Kal Fresubin and 75ml of prune juice each day. This provides him with 50g of protein and 1000 calories each day. Since 28/02/2017 to the last review on 10/01/2018 nothing has changed. The method of administration remains the same i.e. via PEG Bolus. He also has 1000mls of water spread out over the day via bolus.

Extra flushes are required during day and night and his total fluid intake is 2650 mls/24 hour. All fluid and feed given via PEG bolus. Paul is tolerating his feeds very well. PEG site stoma is clean and in good condition.

His nutritional scale is 22 and this shows a high risk; therefore good observation must be adhered to regarding his feeding regimes at all times.

Night report

Paul has a good sleeping pattern. He normally goes to sleep around 9:30pm. He receives lemon wash or sage tea wash at the beginning of the shift to control the excessive sweating during the night. Whole-body embrocation is being rendered followed by the wash. This helps him to relax and get a good night's sleep.

Positioning at night

Paul is on three-hourly positioning as per the positioning protocol using blocks and pillows. Occasionally he asks to change the position after two hours if he doesn't feel comfortable.

Spasms at night

Paul gets strong spasms during the night. When it happens the whole body moves, affecting the positioning as well. His head can come off the pillow or cause hyperextension of the neck, resulting in difficulty in breathing, or the Nippy tubing can be disconnected from the tracheostomy. So, close observation is required and repositioning or head adjustments should be done as and when necessary. The frequency of the spams is much better recently.

Tracheostomy care at night

Tracheostomy care as per the care plan is being given at the beginning of the shift. Secretion is coming out through the stoma as well when he is in bed. So the metalin dressing needs to be changed and stoma should be cleansed at the beginning of the shift without fail. Tracheostomy suction and oral suction should be performed as required. Generally Paul needs an average of 5–6 times suctioning during the night. Inner cannula and green tubing needs changing at least twice during the shift.

Continence at night

Paul is doubly incontinent. However, he has got a regular toileting regime at night. Urine bottle is being offered three hourly during the night with good results. If you ask Paul whether he wants to pass urine or not he is able to tell and he has got moderate capability over his bladder elimination. However, he has no control of his bowel movement yet. Toilet training program continues during the night.

Food and fluid intake and PEG care at night

Paul receives approximately 1000mls of fluids; includes 200mls of Fresubin at 6.00am. His care is being provided as per the PEG care policy.

Physiotherapy

Paul's needs were assessed. He was considered to be at risk of developing chest complications, losing bone mass due to non-weight bearing and losing muscle tone. He had poor head and trunk control.

His physiotherapy sessions included chest physiotherapy, standing on the tilt table for weight bearing with cuff deflation, facial muscle exercise and voice synchronisation. The American Speech-Language-Hearing Association's (ASHA) website explains cuff deflation by saying:

> The main purpose of an inflated tracheotomy tube cuff is to maintain the air delivered from the ventilator to a patient's lungs. The inflated cuff, an internal balloon that surrounds the outer cannula or body of the tracheotomy tube, fills the tracheal space around the tube and prevents breath from escaping through the upper airway. The inflated cuff prevents leakage of air, thereby creating a closed loop between the ventilator and patient and ensuring a consistent delivery of air. However, during periods of cuff inflation, air is not available for phonation or swallowing. The impact on voice, creating aphonia, is immediately evident.

Paul also received gentle passive range of movement exercises for both his upper and lower limb in order to maintain bone and muscle strength. He used a THERA-Trainer (a special exercise bike for people with physical disabilities) which helped the range of movements and joint mobility. His physiotherapy sessions included assistance with neck exercises. He was ventilated using a machine called Nippy-3.

The physiotherapy outcomes were as follows:

Respiration

Paul maintained good ventilation using the Nippy-3+ pressure-controlled ventilator. He was monitored for chest physiotherapy every morning.

The time he was able to tolerate the cuff deflation increased from 20 minutes to more than 40 minutes while standing on the tilt table, without a drop in his oxygen levels. The physiotherapy team worked jointly with the nursing team to monitor the status of Paul's lungs and provided prompt intervention if needed.

Passive Range of Movement (PROM)

Paul tolerated the PROM exercise sessions with little or no complaint of pain. Activities like cycling on THERA-Trainer helped Paul maintain his PROM and also promoted good joint play of lower limb joints.

Paul started practising passive/active assistive neck exercises like rotation of head on either side, tucking of chin in and forward, looking up and down and bending the head on either side. Paul was able to hold head in upright position for an average of five seconds when he is alert and not physically tired. He could not manage longer because his muscles were too weak.

Posture

Paul had low muscle tone in his neck, trunk, upper and lower limbs. However, he showed good symmetry whenever lying, sitting in his wheelchair or standing on the tilt table. When lying down, a single pillow was placed under each knee to prevent him from hyperextending his knees and a hard foam pack was used to keep both ankles in a neutral position. Paul was turned every three hours to the left, on his back and to the right. This was altered if his skin condition or his ventilation needs required this.

Standing

Paul continued to use the tilt table in his standing sessions. In these he maintained good postural alignment and both his ankles were in the appropriate position with suitable support. By the time of discharge, Paul was able to tolerate an average of one hour in a standing position without complaints of pain or discomfort.

Transfers

Paul was unable to weight bear independently. For transfers he used a full body hoist/ceiling tract hoist with the assistance of two people. He required a slide sheet (a special sheet to assist people to move) when he needed to turn or go up and down in the bed.

Treatment at the Raphael Hospital

Recommended input on discharge

When the time comes for Paul's discharge, the physiotherapists recommend that good pulmonary ventilation via bed positioning and oral toileting should be maintained. He should stand in the tilt table at least once a week to maintain the muscle property and bone mass. He should use a THERA-Trainer for cycling to maintain flexibility in his joints and prevent contractures. Cuff deflation should be implemented once a week to maintain pulmonary capacity and active breathing.

Guidelines

The physiotherapy department produced guidelines for the other staff when they needed to position Paul or transfer him. The guidelines for transferring Paul can be seen in Appendix One.

Speech and language therapy (SALT)

Paul's needs were assessed. He required help with communication and swallowing. Swallowing difficulties are known as dysphagia.

Communication

Paul has no acquired language impairment. Since May 2014 he has used a special system on his personal laptop, operating it through a switch set off by movements in his mouth/chin. This software enables Paul to communicate, save messages, access music and the internet, and ultimately allowed him to independently operate machines which had a remote control such as a television once he returned home. Paul said this was difficult to set up, but he uses his chin to spell out words and the computer speaks for him. He likes the system, is able to use the internet, send emails and listen to music, particularly opera. He was asked if the computer was quicker than the spelling system using the alphabet sets and we were told they were the same. Paul is regularly visited by friends and family who communicate with him using alphabet sets, the device on his laptop and, occasionally, lip-reading. Paul Skypes his wife regularly through his laptop computer.

Dysphagia (swallowing difficulties)

Paul is not allowed anything by mouth except for oral trials with a SALT. All nutrition, hydration and medication are provided through a PEG tube, which was placed into his stomach through his abdominal wall.

Paul has severe difficulties with swallowing, known as dysphagia. He has oropharyngeal stage dysphagia, which means that it is difficult for him to use his tongue and jaw due to limited strength and movement. The pharyngeal stage is a combination of voluntary and involuntary control when triggering a swallow: in other words, swallowing involves both conscious and unconscious activity. We are conscious of swallowing when we swallow food or drink but usually unconscious of swallowing saliva. Pharyngeal stage dysphagia for Paul is weak as he has no voluntary control to trigger a swallow and his involuntary swallow trigger is inconsistent. Thus, his severe dysphagia is due to reduced strength together with a limited range of mouth movements. This means Paul is unable to manage his own oral secretions and requires regular oral and chest suction through his tracheostomy tube.

Paul's SALT treatment

Paul's SALT treatment includes Neuro Functional Reorganisational Therapy (NFRT) to improve the oral movements and control to aid in the initial stages of swallowing. This therapy is based on the neurophysiological development of humans and takes people through the various developmental stages.

In June 2015, at Paul's request and following a discussion with the doctor in charge, consent was given for a special treatment. This was carried out under the close supervision of a SALT who had specialised in working with dysphagic patients. Twice weekly Paul was supported by his physiotherapist, his keyworker and his SALT to have synchronized suction for 20 minutes with a special valve developed for patients with a tracheostomy and who required ventilation. Paul was given tastes of whisky during this treatment. Vocalisation and articulation exercises were carried out during these sessions. Daily cuff deflation was also carried out for several minutes to ensure there was some airflow stimulation over the glottis.

Facial expression: Paul began regular exercises for facial expression with the aim of increasing movement in the right side of his face, thus supporting mouth speech as well as oral intake (particularly in relation to lip seal).

Outcome

Dysphagia

Paul's swallowing difficulties improved a little; he was able to achieve full lip seal for three to five seconds and partial lip seal (he has weakness on his right side) for extended periods. His lip seal has been supported in recent sessions with the use of facial tape to increase symmetrical movement. When positioned with his head midline or tilted slightly posteriorly Paul is able to trigger several pharyngeal swallows per session, although not consistently in every session. Paul's ability to swallow remains inconsistent from session to session.

Communication

Paul is able to use mouthing words combined with partner-assisted scanning to maintain communication during sessions. Facial exercises undertaken daily, with his keyworker as well as in physiotherapy and SALT sessions, are aimed at improving oro-motor strength and range of movement. Despite right-sided facial paralysis and left-sided weakness, Paul is able to use facial expression to communicate in context.

Paul became able to achieve vocalisation, such as laughter, on some occasions, for example during sessions with his physiotherapist and SALT, when he was supported to stand in the tilt table and with cuff deflation. He is more likely to be able to vocalise voluntarily when his head is in midline (supported by the physiotherapist) and he is manually assisted to retract his jaw and tilt his head slightly forward.

Recommendations

Paul to be supported by the Raphael Hospital staff or by the community SALT in relation to any issues he may have for his switch-controlled communication system.

Paul to remain *nil by mouth* (except for oral trials) with all nutritional and medicinal requirements supplied through the PEG tube.

He should receive daily chest physiotherapy and be monitored closely for signs of aspiration.

He should have regular cuff deflation, with Passy Muir Valve (PMV) and oral trials of diluted whisky for quality of life (his physiotherapist, SALT and keyworker should be involved in this).

There continues to be an increase in secretions orally and in the pharynx in response to any oral stimulation. With the cuff down for half an hour there is increased risk of aspiration of saliva which may compromise the health of the lungs. It would be prudent to consider a medication for secretion reduction to help this, e.g. hyoscine, glycopyrrolate or atropine.

There will be increased fatigue effect as breathing via the PMV requires some extra respiratory effort. This should be carefully monitored.

Vocalisation/articulation exercises should be carried out during cuff deflation + PMV + oral trials of diluted whisky for pleasure (the physiotherapist, SALT and keyworker should be engaged with these exercises).

Occupational therapy (OT)

The OTs worked together with the physiotherapists. In particular, they wanted to improve Paul's flaccid upper limbs, his lack of voluntary movements, the spasm he experienced when his wrist was extended, his lack of head and neck control and his total dependency for all Activities of Daily Living (ADLs). Their input consisted of physical exercises and positioning of upper limbs. They liaised with specific services regarding any new equipment Paul needed, managed the equipment, kept the family involved and were prepared to help out with any equipment problems when requested.

Outcome

Paul maintained the passive functional ranges in his both upper limbs. The OTs reminded people to refer to the bed positioning guidelines provided by the physiotherapists and said they were involved as necessary with Paul's equipment and positioning needs.

Recommendations

Due to Paul's flaccid upper and lower limbs and poor trunk, head and neck control he requires a tilt-in-space wheelchair. (This is a wheelchair with a feature allowing the whole chair to tilt up to 30 or 60 degrees, depending on the model, while maintaining hip and knee angles at 90 degrees. Paul needed an attendant to propel the chair.) He also required a comfortable chair and a shower commode chair providing appropriate supports, adjustable leg rests, pressure-relieving cushions/surfaces, seat belts, tilt mechanisms and armrests. Paul also needed his arms supported on pillows and they must not dangle over the edge of the chair. When Paul was out in the community, staff should make sure he was comfortably seated in his wheelchair and his head was comfortable too. If necessary, his position should be adjusted.

In anticipation of discharge to home, Paul's community OT organised adaptations for his house with suitable equipment *in situ*. The OTs stressed that all staff working with Paul needed to be aware of how to safely use his equipment and, of course, to follow carefully the transfer procedure when he needed to move into and out of the wheelchair. The principles for the correct seating position can be seen in Appendix Two.

Neuropsychology

The main input from neuropsychology was to undertake a detailed cognitive assessment, to increase Paul's emotional well-being and to improve his overall quality of life.

Paul was seen for one hour a week for assessment and another one hour a week for an individual neuropsychology session to enhance his emotional well-being and quality of life.

Cognitive assessment

Paul completed a detailed assessment. This is reported in Chapter Three. He scored in the above average range on a test estimating premorbid functioning, he had good language skills and was above average on tests of executive functioning. Although he did not have severe memory problems, there were some mild difficulties with visual recognition memory. His basic visual perceptual skills were adequate, although he struggled with some aspects of visual reasoning and visual problem-solving tests (picture completion and Raven's Matrices). This was probably because of eyesight problems: Paul's acuity is poor. He had no problems with a test of mental rotation, which another of our LIS patients, Tracey, found very difficult.

Outcome

Paul was seen by neuropsychology for the purpose of engaging him in activities of his choice with the aim of increasing his emotional well-being and overall quality of life. He chose to work on a wildlife photography project. This involved weekly outings around the grounds of the centre in pursuit of wildlife animals. The photographs were taken by Veronika, then an assistant psychologist at the Raphael Hospital, and later reviewed and discussed with Paul. A collage of the photographs was made to depict the theme of the sessions and Paul chose the way he wanted the photographs to be compiled for the collage. Paul communicated that he enjoyed the sessions and was always coming up with new ideas for what he and the psychologist could look for and photograph. The collage is now on his wall at home.

Recommendations

It is recommended that Paul attends and is supported in available community groups focused around his area of interest (e.g. photography), in order to maintain the continuity of the emotional well-being work carried out by Neuropsychology at the Raphael Hospital. Recently he has been seen for an extra 30 minutes a week to discuss and spell out additions for the current book.

External Applications including Rhythmical Massage and Embrocations

For several years Paul received ongoing treatments with External Applications, Rhythmical Embrocations, Oil Dispersion Bath Therapy and Rhythmical Massage Therapy.

Treatments focussed on managing his spasticity; reducing pain, especially in his neck and shoulder; harmonising left and right-side imbalances; stimulating his breathing activity and reducing congestion; stimulating peripheral circulation, especially to his feet; promoting regular digestion and bowel rhythm; looking after his skin; and reducing episodes of sweating. Paul often expressed his liking and appreciation of these treatments.

The following plans are to establish some continuity at home.

Use of therapeutic oils in home care

In anticipation of Paul's discharge, the use of oil baths at home was discussed with Paul and his wife Liz. The following oils were recommended:

a   for his whole body: Calendula Massage oil by Weleda for whole-body general application any time; aromatherapy oils, including base oils such as olive, almond, calendula, jojoba;
b   for his chest: camphor oil to stimulate and encourage breathing; thyme oil in case of congestion, provided he was not receiving medical treatment; and
c   for his legs; rosemary to stimulate peripheral circulation and help to increase his pulse rate. Liz was asked not to use rosemary if Paul's pulse was above 75/min.

In addition, it was thought that it would be beneficial for Paul to continue receiving Rhythmical Massage Therapy or gentle aromatherapy massage from a trained practitioner.

<u>Skin Care:</u> Paul's skin remained sensitive but was well maintained with regular use of moisturisers and therapeutic oil applications. Paul was pale but well nourished; he experienced sweating episodes.

<u>Warmth:</u> Paul required support to maintain his body warmth. Sometimes his feet became ice cold while he was in his wheelchair, and his shoulder became very cold while he was lying in bed. A foot bath was introduced to maintain warmth in his feet.

Breathing: As noted earlier, Paul was dependent on a portable Nippy-3 ventilator. He showed irregular and insufficient spontaneous breathing and had limited ability to cough, he could, however, occasionally sneeze.

Pulse rate: Paul's pulse rate was regularly observed to be between 50–60 beats per minute. It was noted that previously, when admitted in 2012, he suffered from tachycardia with a rate of 110 beats per minute.

Movements: Tremors and involuntary spasms of the whole body with hip rotating towards the right side and left arm extending were frequently triggered by contact. The left side of Paul's chest and passive movements with the left leg were particularly sensitive to contact. Contact on other areas may also trigger a spasm. After a spasm there was a considerable time period when Paul was able to receive contact on those areas without starting another spasm.

Art therapy

Paul was interested in the arts, having been a photographer and an opera singer. He was also good at languages and eager to learn about new things. His needs were considered to be: greater social interaction, emotional support and well-being, self-confidence, self-worth and sense of identity, and help with the lack of movement in his hands. The art therapy sessions involved Paul interacting with the art therapist; talking about art and acknowledging feelings and emotions that may arise through art; encouragement to decide on motif, colours, techniques and materials he wished the art therapist to use; and using hand over hand to provide passive movement when painting.

His chosen project was 'Sweeney Todd', a fictional Victorian character. Use was made of collages, watercolour painting, drawing cut-outs, sponges and other materials. For some of the techniques, hand-over-hand support was provided so that Paul could have the most immediate experience when engaging with his chosen media. In the next stage, Paul added writing and cut-outs to the mixed media collage of his Sweeney Todd project. He made clear his instructions and was well able to express his ideas on the progress of his artwork. It seemed easy for him to imagine the possible outcomes when deciding on each technique. He appeared to enjoy explaining his plans, thoughts and reflections when conversing with the therapist and often employed humour to convey his message. When Paul finished the Sweeney Todd project, it was framed and displayed in his home. It was felt that his confidence and belief in himself as an artist had increased as a result of completing such an impressive piece of work.

Paul then decided to continue work on a painting he had started some time ago but had never finished. He asked the art therapist to carry on with a watercolour painting of a tiger in a jungle. The colours used were carefully selected and directed by Paul. Humour was always a vital means of expression for him throughout the creative process. For example, he asked the therapist to give the tiger lipstick to give another dimension to the meaning of the painting.

Recommendations

Paul seemed to make good use of the time and space provided to express himself and to continue to develop as an artist. Given his personal background as a professional photographer, actor and singer, integrating the creative arts was essential for Paul's emotional, mental and physical well-being. It is important not to deny the value of this for Paul, not only in terms of emotional support and self-expression but also for his self-confidence and sense of identity. It is recommended that he continues to engage in artistic activities as well as psychological therapies to ensure his overall well-being and good quality of life.

Music therapy

It was hoped that music therapy would improve Paul's communication, social interaction and emotional well-being. The aims were to provide opportunities for Paul to engage in music within a group; to provide opportunities for Paul to be able to choose songs to engage with; and to encourage Paul to mouth words to songs to support his communication, interaction and emotional well-being.

Outcome

Paul attended music therapy regularly. He engaged well with the therapists and appeared to enjoy musical interaction. He chose what he wanted to work on and fed back his views using mouthed words and communication strategies. He provided the therapy team with a number of lists of artists he enjoys and supports the structure of the session through choice making and mouthing words. This supports his sense of musical self and self within the group – creating a number of roles, including observer, director, musician and audience member. It is, in our opinion, useful for Paul to attend the group to explore his musical preferences and to share within a group situation.

Discharge plan

Attending the music therapy group offered Paul the opportunity to support and reflect the important access to musical interaction and shared expression that he has at home – with societies, close friends and choirs. We hope that he will continue to have access to these opportunities once home. Any support with attending these groups would be highly recommended and we suggest for Paul to continue to attend and support performance groups where possible. If this is not possible we would recommend attendance of music-based social groups to aid in his access to creativity-based social interaction and expression using musical choice, lyric and reminiscence.

These summaries are included to give an idea of the everyday treatment received by Paul and, indeed, by many of the patients at the Raphael Hospital (see for example, *Surviving Brain Injury after Assault: Gary's Story* [Wilson et al. 2016]). All patients, even those in a vegetative state, receive regular therapy.

8 Interviews with Paul's friends

Barbara Hunter – friend from church

When Paul and Liz were going to be married they came to my church and then came to my home group at my house with some other people. During that time I got to know them and I went to their wedding, and from there on we became good friends. Paul was always very much "there" in our home group; a great talker, he was always leading us off on tangents all sorts of things and Liz was always bringing him back again. He was a wonderful chap and everyone loved him. On one occasion he took a wonderful photo of the entire group which he gave to one of our ladies, Betty, who had to move. She always had it by her bed, the picture he took; that was the kind of man he was. He was very kind and I know he did other wonderful things within the church, but he certainly enriched our group. And we went to different things to hear him singing and became part of his and Liz's life. So when he had the stroke we were all devastated. There was no thought that we wouldn't be with him. We always think about him in our group, we always pray for him and we visit him and we keep in contact with Liz. We have been on the journey with Paul. First of all we were so devastated, we did not know what was going to happen, but gradually we have been encouraged as we have seen him at Raphael improving and always so upbeat. We don't see the sad side I am sure he must have. When I see him he always has a joke for me – it might be a bit rude, it might not – and I write it down as he blinks it. He always has a joke for me and we have a nice rapport really. I have known him for over 17 years. I found out about the stroke as Liz came round to see me – we didn't know how serious it was at that time – and from then on I visited him frequently. It was shattering to see him in ICU; we didn't know what was going to happen. We thought he was going to go to another place at first, Putney, and we thought "Oh no", but he went to the Raphael Hospital – that was the very best thing for him. The relationship we have is due to our faith, which is very important to us, as it is to Paul and Liz. When Paul finally comes home we aim to have the home group at his and Liz's home so that Paul can once again be a part of it.

Iona and John Jenkins – Iona was Paul's singing teacher

Being a singing teacher I used to do charity concerts and some of my pupils sang in other groups. I had heard Paul sing several times but I hadn't met him. Then I phoned and asked him if he would be willing to take part in one of my concerts and he was overjoyed. We had about four good singers but he was the best of all my singers. He was the best entertainer of all my singers. He was so good-looking and engaged with the audience and moved around and liked to dress up. I had another singer who was also a tenor and he had the most beautiful voice, but he didn't entertain like Paul. Over the years we grew to love Paul very much; he became like my son. Lovely, lovely man. So enthusiastic, never stopped talking; sometimes we had to say, "Right then, that's enough Paul." I say to him now I can't wait until you can speak again and I keep saying to him for goodness sake breathe, if you can breathe you can take that thing from your throat and we can hear you speak and hear you sing and he can eat. I am hoping it will happen; I think he wants to sing again. Of course he became part of the family. John's sister-in-law came to all his concerts and he came to all our family meetings. He hadn't fulfilled all his potential as a singer when he had the stroke. We have come down the Raphael to do concerts for Paul, the patients and families and Paul loves it. He mouths along to all the songs. We love performing and we love coming to do the concerts for Paul and for the others, as I am sure they get something from it. We heard the day after [it happened] *from Liz that Paul had his stroke. The night before he had been talking to me as he was really depressed, as the builders had messed up his conservatory in the other house, and he said he had had a terrible headache all day and hadn't been well and so I am guessing the stroke was already starting. I am not saying the stress caused the stroke, but I am sure it didn't help. We went to see him two days later in hospital and we went straight past him, we didn't recognise him – it was so upsetting. On reflection he didn't look like he looks now. We don't think of that now, he is still Paul; it doesn't matter what he looks like, he is still Paul. The amazing thing is that before the stroke if Paul made a mistake with one of his songs or did something wrong he would be so cross with himself and get so depressed, and now he isn't depressed at all as far as we know. He is full of it. I just wish he could talk, not as much as before* [laughter], *but there is so much he wants to say but it is so slow. But he was always part of my group after that first concert, he was one of my main forces.*

Keith and Barbara Payne

[Keith] *Paul tends to do things with quite a bang. He arrived in about 1984 into our lives in one of Barbara's shows,* Bless the Bride, *where he played Thomas Trout. He was in shows, he performed, he contributed to the world and our world and we became friends with him and his then wife Sue. He had an eye for detail: he would make cakes, do loft ladders, but never did mine because he just ran out of time – I still nag him about that now. He was a very talented man, very particular in all he did. We went on a holiday on the Thames in 1987 on a riverboat, it was fairly archaic for various reasons and Paul's boat skills are nowhere near as good as his cake-making or decorating or building skills. His primary skill which remains to this day is to deliver words in a certain order and a lot of them – we miss that. He was the most lively, gregarious, into everything person, which is still there inside his shell, we know that. When we come to visit him we are still as irreverent with him and he back to us as ever we were. I remember once when once of his friends got married and he was the wedding photographer. He was in the transition phase from his job in the metropolitan police and his motorbike. We mustn't forget his motorbike. He used to have a motorbike which he was knocked off at times by people and he had a view on that. At the friend's wedding he had taken all the pictures and we were back at their house sat down with Liz at a table in the bottom of the garden. I phoned Paul on his mobile and said, "Is that Paul Allen?" and he said, "Yes, can I help you?" and I said, "Would you please come and talk to your wife as she has been here for 45 minutes?" I don't know how long they had been married at that point, but Liz didn't know the couple that had married very well and Paul just went off and was yak, yak, yak. This was Paul, he would talk for England. In Chislehurst at his operatic societies' auctions, we would be sitting in his house and he would have his many records and CDs, which he loved, and the goods would be passed round the room to be auctioned. He would be sat one side of the room and I the other. I would frequently pick up two or three of his CDs and they would go round the room, and when they got to Paul he would say "I have got this one" and bid on it. Of course the whole room would be in hysterics.*

[Barbara] *Going back I was asked* [to take part in a production] *by Sue, his first wife, who also performed and directed. It was out at Streatham Hill, which is where she worked, and she was doing a production of* Orpheus and the Underworld. *The woman who was playing Cupidon was either ill or had dropped out and she* [Sue] *asked me if I would go along and play the role, which I did. Paul was also in the production and all I can remember throughout the rehearsal is her screaming out, asking Paul to shut up. I know we all say it but he really did talk for England, and he still does – he* is incredible. *Every time Paul does a wedding, is singing, doing photography, attending events, he is off yakking somewhere. This is why it was so devastating when Paul had his stroke. It was like a death knell to us, and certainly because my husband (Keith) is of a similar age to Paul it really hit him very hard – there but for the grace of God.*

[Keith] *I had fear when I had to go and see him first, terrified. I didn't know how to talk to him, didn't know if he was there.*

[Barbara] *I couldn't talk to him the very first time when he came home and was in the back garden I couldn't cope.*

[Liz] *I have always tried to be there when people first saw Paul, and even now I try to be there to help with the communication to read his lips.*

[Barbara] *Obviously we have got used to it now but that very first time it was so emotional.*

[Keith] *I burst into tears, it is so frightening. It is not his fault, it is us struggling to cope to make sense of it, but it is still Paul, he is still all there. When we first saw him he wasn't, he had no sort of movement.*

[Barbara] *But he was still there. But now it is easier to see the sparkle to see what he is communicating, the sparkle in his eye. You can tell when he is telling a joke, his face tells it, he has much more expression in his face. We still find it difficult as we don't know the routine, the blocks, like Liz does. She knows it so quickly – we still have to think.*

Eric Seers – colleague in police force

Although we worked for the same organisation (Metropolitan Police), I actually first met Paul through amateur operatics in 1985. We both auditioned for the same part in a show. Paul was given the part over me (good decision) but we got on well together. Then in the early 90s we came to work on the same project for the police which lasted for many years. Because of our different positions our relationship there was mostly just work related. But in the same decade we performed together in many operettas/musicals and continued to do so in the following decade. Our social interaction was more prevalent in that field rather than work.

    Paul is a very proud man; proud of what he's done and proud of his achievements. To that end he always sets the bar high. Perfection, style and individuality are key to him meeting his objectives. He pushed himself hard when he put his mind to something.

    I heard of Paul's condition soon after he'd suffered the stroke. My reaction was naturally one of shock. Although I had not seen him for several months I knew him to be fit and comparatively young in his mid-50s. When I became aware of the severity of his condition I went to see him on my own just after he'd moved to the Raphael Hospital. That was very difficult; we had no communication, all I could do was talk to Paul with no reaction coming back from him. Soon after, I went again with a work colleague and gradually in the next few months we learnt the alphabet system used to communicate with Paul. In those early months Paul also developed some movement with the left side of his mouth which allowed him to make some facial expressions and so our communication improved considerably. Since those early months four of us, all former work colleagues, visit him (two at a time) on an informal rota every Thursday afternoon.

Our relationship now is a bit like a few mates meeting up for a beer and a chat – and I think it's important he has that social interaction. Despite his severe physical limitations his mind is fully operational and alert. He keeps abreast of world events and news, follows sport and has an opinion on any subject we care to mention. But what makes our meetings so easy is his attitude. He is always positive, always upbeat, always has something to say (that's the Paul we've always known!) and always interested in what we have to say – a good bit of "man chat" with the odd joke thrown in. We usually spend an hour and a half with him and there's never a moment of embarrassed silence. In fact, we're usually going full flow when our meetings are brought to an end by the arrival of a physio and nurse ready to take him off for a therapy session. One thing is certain from our conversations – Paul's devotion to and love for Liz and his desire to return home on a permanent basis. The care he receives at the Raphael Hospital is second to none and it must be a credit to them that Paul is still with us. The Raphael has been active in supporting Paul's desire to return home but there appears to be an impasse with his local authority in providing an appropriate care package to support this. I know this is a big disappointment and frustration to both Paul and Liz.

Dave Morgan – colleague in police force

I first met him, I think, in 1986 when I joined a small team doing computer procurement for the Metropolitan Police. He was always talking! We had a sign on a stick that we held up sometimes, it said SHUT UP PAUL. *We challenged him once to see how long he could keep quiet – he lasted two minutes! Because we moved between different departments we only saw each other occasionally until we both worked on the CRIS project. In 2000 we were outsourced to an American company and we then worked together, finally ending up in The Royal Courts of Justice in the Strand. Just the two of us worked in an office answering phone calls for two years until one day I* told him that I was taking early retirement six months later and I wanted him to be the first to know. He stayed working in different roles for the company for a few more years.

Paul was always very thorough in everything that he did. He was painstaking in the work he did on his Victorian house, trying to get it back to its original state. Rather than replace balustrades on his porch with new ones from Wickes or B&Q he removed a good one and had copies made in the same design. I found that he was always trying to do three things at once, rushing from one place to the next. An uncle at his wedding told me, "The trouble with Paul is that wherever he is, he's supposed to be somewhere else"! He loved doing his operatic roles and was a member of several groups. After a performance he would be on a high, but a few days later would be depressed and start rehearsing another role. He admitted to me that he was quite shy, but when singing he would take on the role so that it wasn't him. He would never stand up in front of a group of people and do a talk – that would be himself, and not playing a role.

I heard about the stroke I think within a few days. It was a while before I visited him, and although warned, it was a shock to see him in that state. Four of his old colleagues try to visit in pairs every week, although this is not always possible. It's hard to believe that Paul has been in this state for five years now.

9   Paul's continuing involvement with music

In April 2017 a concert to celebrate Paul was organised by his friends. This included his ex-wife who was travelling from Malaga, Spain where she now lives. Paul had not seen some of the people attending the concert for 30 years. He spelt out that the friends told the story of his musical life through song. He said it was superb and very moving. There was a storyteller who was excellent. The first song was from *The Pirates of Penzance*. There were some opera singers there who sang things Paul used to sing. Liz said that there were loads of people there who had known him for years and they made a CD of the concert. This was comprised of a number of photographs taken over the course of the concert.

In May Paul went to Covent Garden Opera House in London. He and Liz went by a taxi especially adapted to take wheelchairs. The journey took about two hours each way. He told us that Catherine Jenkins and Alfie Bow were performing; they sang for three hours and they were both superb.

On one occasion Paul spelt out his three favourite musical memories. In his words these were: *(1) When I was in my 20s I sang with the choir of King's College in Cambridge Cathedral. (2) In my 30s I played the pirate king in* The Pirates of Penzance. *I was in a cast of 60 and the audience numbered 1,100. This was also my first professional part. (3) When I was 51 and for two consecutive years I sang at The Royal Albert Hall.* He added, *Over the years, I have sung in Latin, Italian, German, French, Welsh and sometimes English.*

He also wanted to talk about his cycling. He said: *For 29 years I was a very keen biker. I commuted to work every day and my longer trips included Scotland, Wales and the west country. I also went on several bike tours of European countries, one of which was 4,500 miles. I was 28 years old. Five of us did the trip together. We rode as far east as Yugoslavia, as far south as mainland Greece and Corfu, and as far north as Switzerland. I bought my first motorbike when I was 17 years old but I did not take to four wheels*

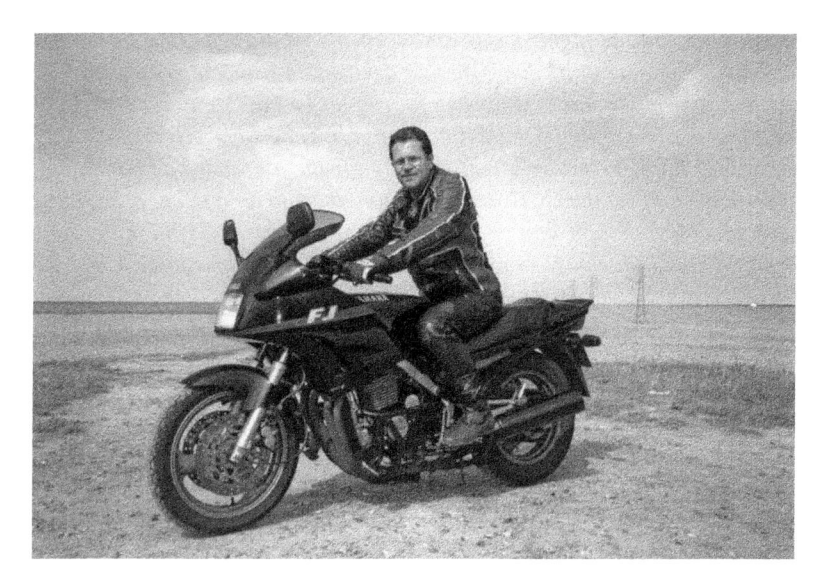

Figure 9.1 Paul on his motorcycle.

until seven years later. However, I was driving until I had the stroke and I am still the proud owner of a beautiful Mercedes E class (Figure 9.1).

Paul was meant to leave the Raphael Hospital and return home by the end of June 2016, but this did not happen. He and Liz were waiting for continuing health care (CHC) from his local authority to provide money for the care package. Both are angry with the CHC.

Liz said, *In May 2016 I received a phone call from the funder from the clinical commissioning group (CCG), saying she was preparing Paul's home care package. Her first offer was for one carer. I explained that Paul needed two carers, day and night. She said, "We don't do that in Bromley." I explained that Paul needed to be hoisted and one person could not do it safely. She then offered to send a person in a couple of times a day to help with hoisting. I pointed out that he may empty his bowels any time, and if the "extra" person had already been then he would just have to sit until that extra person came back. She then said we could have another person but they would have to live in and be available for night time as well as day. She was still adamant that Bromley would not provide two night carers, that Paul would be put in position at about 11pm and would be fine until the next morning. She also said Paul could have a special air mattress, even though we had been told he cannot have that type of mattress.*

The next phone call was much the same, with the refusal to allow Paul to be turned in the night. I was asked when I would like Paul home and was given the date of 21 June. We had decided on which agency we would use and a group of ladies were sent to train to be Paul's carers. They were nice ladies but totally unsuitable for the job. They were given three days to train at Raphael but were really wrong for the job; they had no nursing experience and yet the CCG were expecting them to do nursing procedures such as cuff deflation and changing his tracheostomy. As the date drew nearer, I could see that it would be unsafe for Paul to come home. I sent the CCG representative an email saying it was not safe at that time and it would be good to meet at the Raphael on 1 July. No physiotherapy had been organised or any other therapy. I had previously asked her to come and meet Paul but she just said, "I don't need to, I have read his report."

She did come to Raphael but would not budge from saying Bromley does not allow people to have two night carers and he would be put in position at night and stay there till the next morning, and "There were a lot of people with Paul's condition in Bromley". She also said she had spoken with Dr Lal and he agreed with her. Paul spelt out, "I don't want to go home to die, I will stay here." She just said "Okay, it's your decision" and left the room. She did not speak to his carers or watch how he was handled and hoisted into his chair or bed. The manager of the agency was also present throughout.

Paul said that *the CCG representative was stubborn* and added a comment we will not repeat here. Egan thinks the file on his care package is closed but he hopes she will persuade the CHC to reopen it.

When asked to describe the main ways that the LIS had affected him, Paul said it made him use his brain more and he now writes more. He did not write before this happened and now he has a book about his experiences in press. "What have you learnt?" we said to Paul. He thought he had become a better person, more considerate and more patient. "Are there any positives from having LIS?", we inquired. *Yes,* said Paul, *self-assessment has improved and I now have a granddaughter.* He was asked, too, what message he would like to give to other survivors of LIS. He replied, *Don't give up, keep trying.* When asked how he saw the future Paul said that he was going to recover or else become an author. He also wanted to be able to sing solo again. He said he felt his brain was getting better as he had learnt a few words in 26 languages. When asked what he feared he said he feared *that he would not recover*. He was asked what he thought about when he was in his room alone. He replied that he thought *about concerts and had also designed a big house for himself with a music room, a home cinema and a swimming pool*. He said he sang in his head and said that he could remember all the parts he had sung and everyone else's parts too. Paul's sense of humour still shines through: he once blinked out that he was changing his name to Lucky!

For a while Paul stopped having music therapy at the RMC but he communicated that he wanted to have it again. The therapy consisted of the music therapist seeing Paul on a one-to-one basis and playing music and songs of Paul's choice. This was fed back to the music therapist who said that Paul was on his radar, so the therapy sessions recommenced. Paul now sees the new music therapist, Michael, once a week. They have certain things in common, notably an Irish background, and both say that *Sweeney Todd* is their favourite show. Paul told us that he played the part of Sweeney Todd 20 years ago in the Bob Hope Theatre.

In one of our weekly sessions, Paul was told about Rosemary Johnson, once a violinist with the Welsh National Opera Orchestra. Following a terrible car accident which left her unable to move or speak, Miss Johnson had not played for 29 years until a project between Plymouth University and The Royal Hospital for Neuro-Disability, Putney linked her brain to a computer using Brain Computer Music Interfacing software. This allowed her to compose and play music again through sending her thoughts to a colleague she had last played with before the car accident (*The Telegraph*, 22 August 2017). We contacted Professor Eduardo Miranda at Plymouth University to ask if something similar could be developed for Paul to enable him to "sing" again. Professor Miranda replied saying he thought it might be possible, but a sponsor would be required to provide something in the region of £65,000. Meanwhile, we should contact him again in six months' time to see how the project was developing. When this information was fed back to Paul to see how he felt about the project, his first communication was that he would rather sing himself. What if that isn't possible, he was asked. He then blinked out, *Would you sing for me?* He asked this of Barbara Wilson, who cannot sing in tune! He was assumed to be joking and was told he should find someone who can sing well! We then discussed the possibility of raising money and Paul thought a concert might work. He was requested to discuss this with Liz. We have just contacted Professor Eduardo again as we have just reached the six months deadline. We await a reply.

10 Quality of life for people with LIS, and assessing capacity

The World Health Organisation (WHO) propose that quality of life (QoL) is

> an individual's perception of his or her position in life in the context of the culture and value systems in which they live and in relation to their goals, expectations, standards and concerns. It is a broad ranging concept affected in a complex way by the person's physical health, psychological state, personal beliefs, social relationships and the relationship to salient features of their environment.
>
> (The WHOQoL Group 1995)

In considering this proposition of QoL in the context of a significant, chronic disability such as LIS, it could be argued that a positive adjustment to the disability would be indicative of a good QoL. However, it could equally be argued that it is not possible for an individual diagnosed with LIS to have a high QoL due to the significant levels of physical disability.

It is a challenge to define the term "quality of life" (QoL), as it can have a different meaning for each individual which can lead to corresponding personal definitions. Often in health and social care settings QoL is regarded in terms of health. The conception of QoL can be traced back to the 1940s when the WHO defined health as a "state of complete physical, mental and social well-being, and not merely the absence of disease and infirmity" (WHO 1947). However, the utilisation of the term "well-being" has led to confusion and disagreement about what is health and what is QoL. Such confusion can be seen throughout the medical literature where there appears to be a common understanding that good QoL suggests being in good health and experiencing subjective well-being and life satisfaction (Goode 1994). This gives rise to the question: can someone diagnosed with a significant disability such as LIS have good QoL given the impact of their diagnosis on health? Whilst arguably health is one of the most important domains of overall QoL, other domains exist and are key to an individual's QoL. These domains include

Quality of life for people with LIS, and assessing capacity   69

employment, education, housing, environment, cultural values, spirituality and so on. Having such a vast array of domains when considering overall QoL adds to the complexity of definition and measurement. What can be agreed on is that QoL is important to everyone. It is a multifaceted paradigm that relies on subjective appraisals of negative and positive characteristics of life.

Understanding QoL and the elements in QoL in LIS is important as it has implications for care management, ethical issues and intervention. However, it has been argued that communication limitations make QoL assessments in LIS patients difficult (Murrell 1999). It is claimed that this issue has affected the day-to-day assessment of QoL in people with LIS despite the advent and subsequent use of communication aids and devices. In the case of Paul, assessment is not hampered by him having LIS as he has a very clear and helpful communication system (as mentioned in Chapter Six), the only issue being the length of time it takes to utilise this system.

Over the last decade the issue of QoL in LIS has been explored, and interestingly reported QoL appears to be similar to that of healthy people and patients with non-terminal chronic disease (e.g. Bruno et al. 2011; Laureys et al. 2007; Lulé et al. 2009; Rousseau et al. 2015; Moons et al., 2006); and better than that of those with terminal cancer (McGee et al. 1991).

Lulé and colleagues (2009) report an unpublished study (Ghorbel et al., unpublished) in which patients with LIS were assessed, indicating that their subjective QoL was not related to physical impairment nor could it be predicted by this factor. These reports suggest that individuals with LIS maintain a positive QoL despite their significant physical limitations. This was indeed true of Tracey, described in Chapter Three (Wilson and Okines 2014). This could be due in part to factors of QoL previously noted in studies of severe disability which include disability status, family and social support, use of medical devices and levels of depression (Rousseau et al. 2011; 2013; 2015).

Doble and colleagues (2003) reported that such findings are seen as incongruous to many healthy individuals and medical professionals who might assume that the QoL of a LIS patient is so limited that life may not be worth living. Indeed, Kubler and colleagues (2005) reported that when significant others were asked to evaluate the QoL of a patient with severe motor impairment, arguably akin to LIS, they rated a significantly lower QoL than did the patients themselves. Ganzini and Block (2002) suggest such a dichotomy may be due to a psychological defence mechanism in that healthy people may find it difficult to imagine the experiences and emotions of severely impaired patients. This contradiction can be classed as the "disability paradox"; in other words, why is it that many people with serious and persistent disabilities, such as LIS, report that they experience a good or excellent QoL when those around them perceive them as living an undesirable daily existence? (Albrecht and Devlieger 1999).

Those studies which have considered QoL in LIS have indicated that people diagnosed with LIS report positive QoL. However, none of these studies have considered changes in QoL over time. Arguably what is equally important to understand is whether QoL is only situation and time specific (i.e. at the point of assessment) or is it longitudinal (i.e. stable over time)? The only study to date that has considered this question was conducted by Rosseau and colleagues (2015). They surveyed people with LIS over a six-year period with the aim of determining the contribution of social demographic and clinical factors in predicting stability of QoL over time. The findings of this study concurred with other studies exploring QoL in LIS, showing that people with LIS report good and satisfactory QoL. The authors were able to show that QoL remains stable over time.

In order to understand how Paul perceives his QoL he was asked to complete the Short Form-36 (SF-36 – Ware et al. 1993) as well as to provide qualitative information about QoL. The SF-36 is a 36-item questionnaire which measures QoL across eight domains. The domains are both physically and emotionally based and are as follows: physical functioning; role limitations due to physical health; role limitations due to emotional problems; energy/fatigue; emotional well-being; social functioning; pain; general health. The SF-36 includes a single item that identifies perceived change in health. The inclusion of this item enables clinicians to use the SF-36 to assess change over time and treatment. Significant numbers of published studies have demonstrated its capabilities as a global QoL measure, leading to it having been widely validated for numerous patient groups including LIS.

On the SF-36 Paul unsurprisingly showed maximal limitations in physical activities (all scores were zero). He felt his general health was good, he believed he was functioning well and he gained benefit from social interaction. He did not rate himself as having any emotional problems and indicated overall that he had a positive QoL (see Table 10.1)

Although Paul's scores are in line with many of the studies investigating QoL in LIS with regard to physical well being, there are some differences in other areas as reported by, for example, Leplege and colleagues (1998), in which they compared results from SF-36 from LIS patients with age-matched controls. LIS patients, like Paul, predictably showed maximal limitations in physical activities and reported significant limitations in usual role activities because of health problems. However, unlike Paul, they reported restrictions in social functioning due to physical or emotional problems. Paul reports that his physical limitations may have impacted on him accessing social activities, as he has to rely on others

Table 10.1 Paul's scores from SF-36

Domain	Score
Physical functioning	0.0
Role functioning/physical	0.0
Role functioning/emotional	66.7
Energy/fatigue	70.0
Emotional well-being	76.0
Social functioning	75.0
Pain	100.0
General health	90.0
Health change	—

to facilitate access, but emotionally he believes LIS does not limit his social activities. The LIS patients assessed by Leplege and colleagues also showed significant limitations in usual role activities because of emotional problems and scored significantly less on the vitality items (dealing with energy and fatigue). Interestingly, Paul perceives his energy and fatigue as in line with those around him. He does not believe he has less energy than prior to his stroke and believes that it is simply used in different ways. In terms of mental health (i.e. emotional well-being) the patients with LIS, as with Paul, all scored consistently with the control group, suggesting that a diagnosis of LIS is not a precursor to mental health limitations. When considering Paul, he is a balanced person with no obvious depression, anxiety or other mood issues despite the severe limitations placed on him because of his diagnosis of LIS. This is not to say he does not get frustrated or low in mood at times, but this is mainly because he is still in hospital and the funders of his placement are not providing the financial and physical support he needs to return to his home with his wife. This does not however impact on his daily QoL.

Upon meeting Paul, it is apparent he is happy with his life. He is rarely seen without a smile (although this is a partial smile because of his paralysis) and he is eager to interact with those around him, often using humour to engage people. He is always patient with those who are unable to use his communication system and talks openly and frankly about his emotions and experiences. He reports that he sees his QoL as one that is positive and provides opportunities for learning and development.

To conclude the section on QoL, people with LIS appear to believe life is worth living despite their diagnosis, and despite what others around them perceive their QoL to be. In the case of Paul, he has reported he believes his life is worth living and those around him can see he evidently enjoys life and this has appeared to have been stable since his admission to the Raphael Hospital.

Assessing capacity for people who are locked-in

Neuropsychologists and other staff in the UK are sometimes asked to make judgements as to whether or not people have capacity. This is as a result of the Mental Capacity Act of 2005.

The Mental Capacity Act

The Mental Capacity Act (2005) provides a code of practice that healthcare professionals in the UK should adhere to when working with or caring for patients who lack capacity to make decisions for themselves.

Capacity should be assessed in the context of a specific decision, as patients may have capacity in some circumstances but not others; for example, they may have capacity to decide whether or not they will take antibiotics but not capacity to manage their own financial affairs. In cases where it is judged there is a temporary loss of capacity and that full capacity can reasonably be expected to return, only decisions which are time critical should be taken. The options considered around capacity should be the least restrictive to the patient's rights. It can only be determined that a patient lacks capacity after all reasonable efforts to enable the patient to make a decision have been exhausted. It should not be assumed that the patient lacks capacity when the decision that they take appears to be unwise.

The Mental Capacity Act sets out five core principles:

1. A person is assumed to have capacity. A lack of capacity has to be clearly demonstrated.
2. No one should be treated as unable to make a decision unless all practicable and reasonable steps to help him or her have been exhausted and shown not to work.
3. A person is entitled to make an unwise decision. This does not necessarily mean they lack capacity.
4. If it is decided a person lacks capacity then any decisions taken on their behalf must be in their best interests.
5. Any decision taken on behalf of a person who lacks capacity must take into account their rights and freedom of action. Any decision/action must show consideration of the least restrictive options or intervention possible to meet need.

In order to assess capacity, the Act details a two-stage test that must be followed:

1. **The diagnostic test:** Does the person have an impairment, or a disturbance in the functioning, of their mind or brain? This can include,

for example, conditions associated with mental illness, concussion, or symptoms of drug or alcohol abuse.
2   **The functional test:** Does the impairment or disturbance mean that the person is unable to make a specific decision when they need to? In this part of the test all appropriate and practical support must be offered to the patient before continuing on. This may include ensuring all documentation is in the first language of the patient, that documentation is both visual and verbal and, in the case of someone with LIS, appropriate communication aids and/or communication experts are part of the assessment.

This functional part of the test establishes that, to be able to make a decision, a person should be able to:

1   Understand information relevant to the decision.
2   Retain the information – they have to be able to retain the information given for long enough to make the decision. There is no set time limit prescribed for this.
3   Use or weigh that information as part of the process of making the decision.
4   Communicate their decision. A person is deemed as not having capacity if they are unable to communicate.

The Mental Capacity Act recognises LIS as a possible exception, acknowledging that people with LIS can in fact still understand, retain and use information and so would not be regarded as lacking capacity in these three areas. However, they note that some people with LIS can communicate by blinking an eye, whereas others cannot communicate at all. *Therefore, those that can communicate would not be regarded as lacking capacity, whereas those who cannot would be classed as lacking capacity.*

Assessing mental capacity in LIS

As previously acknowledged throughout this book, individuals with LIS are extremely physically impaired but have intact consciousness, hearing and normal or near to normal cognitive abilities (Smith and Delargy 2005). However, they require those around them to facilitate communication and without this they would be effectively "imprisoned". Being without a "voice" means people with LIS are disempowered and have no ability to make decisions around their care and future life. It is more common now that people are preparing advance directives and informing their loved ones as to what they would wish to happen in the case of severe illness or accident. However, arguably it would be difficult for many of us to predict what we would want to happen if we were "locked-in". It has been highlighted that families often experience high levels of distress in dealing with treatment decisions when faced with a loved one having been diagnosed with LIS, despite that person being able to process information (Maiser et al. 2016).

There is empirical evidence suggesting that patients with LIS may have retained the capacity to make decisions about their care, their future needs and treatment (e.g. Carrington and Birns 2012). However, given the patient's limited responsiveness it can be assumed by healthcare professionals that the patient is cognitively impaired and therefore unable to participate in their own healthcare decisions. Such assumption is arguably dangerous and has many ethical implications, especially in use of life-prolonging treatments such as the use of gastrostomy and tracheostomy, or end-of-life care. Given the families' distress and the difficulty for the healthcare professional in the context of decision making it is imperative that that healthcare professionals prioritise communication rehabilitation right from the point of diagnosis. Making communication rehabilitation the priority will empower the person with LIS to participate fully in all decision making and, in turn, will support families and healthcare professionals at those points when assessing the patient's mental capacity is required.

The Mental Capacity Act states that all patients making decisions regarding their healthcare should be facilitated to understand all relevant information and to express their views. In the case of LIS there is a paucity of evidence to support healthcare professionals through the ethical quagmire of managing such complex cases. It is imperative that a thorough neurological, neuropsychological and communication assessment is conducted as soon as possible after diagnosis, and indeed throughout the person with LIS's life, in order to understand their preserved cognitive abilities and enable them to participate fully in their decisions.

As has been highlighted in this book, Paul has been "enabled" to communicate using a communication system that is individual to him. He expresses to those who work with him that this is his "voice" for this current time and he uses it well. His wish would be to be able to express himself verbally, i.e. using his own voice. There have been many times in working with Paul where establishing his mental capacity for decisions has been important, not only for decisions in his day-to-day care but also for major decisions around where he wishes to live, who should support him with his finances and his wishes around end-of-life care.

Assessment of Paul's capacity over decisions has followed a clear framework which has included neuropsychological assessment, current assessment of his physical well-being (i.e. no presence of infection which in turn may affect his cognition), choosing the best time of day (usually late morning), involving one of his keyworkers who is very familiar with his communication aid, and ensuring enough time is allocated (given his communication is very slowed using his aid). If required, Paul is provided with visual aids placed in his eyeline. For more complex decisions the capacity will be assessed over a number of occasions at different times of day (e.g. the decision around his preferred place to live). This is important as he can tire easily, and this in turn affects his ability to communicate, and the 'listener' may not be sure they have understood his communication. Paul is always patient and accepting when the therapist turns up once again to go through the capacity assessment.

In many of situations when capacity needs to be established for Paul there has been no difficulty at all and the decision has not been a challenge. However, in the case of where he wants to live, he wants to be able to return to his own home. While establishing his capacity to make this decision was not difficult, ensuring his wishes are met has been, and still is, an ethical, political and clinical quagmire.

One more measure to illustrate that Paul feels his QoL is reasonable is his response to Seligman's (2011) PERMA model (**P**ositive emotion, **E**ngagement, **R**elationships, **M**eaning and **A**chievement). He communicated that he felt "positive" about life, he was "engaged" and gave as an example the fact that he had designed a house for himself in some detail. For "relationships" Paul said he had received more than 120 visitors since coming to the Raphael Hospital. He felt his life had "meaning" because he had sung in 60 shows. For "achievement" he reminded us that he was co-author of this book and was also writing another book about his life.

In conclusion, LIS is a rare and serious condition presenting with profound motor deficits and presumed intact cognition. As a result, it brings about communication challenges. Such challenges can affect the understanding of the decision-making process in individuals with LIS and these must be addressed by a clear framework as to how to assess capacity in such individuals. As has been reported in this book, research indicates that many individuals with LIS report that they have a good QoL and feel happy. Therefore, it is important that communication rehabilitation is prioritised from the point of diagnosis, rather than making assumptions about perceived QoL, in order to ensure the person with LIS can participate in decisions around their life choices. Continued assessment and discussions should take place with the person with LIS in order to ensure their wishes are considered. In taking such an approach, establishing capacity should not be difficult in those diagnosed with LIS.

11 Ethical issues in LIS

It is difficult to imagine being paralysed, unable to speak while remaining fully aware, yet this is the life of a person diagnosed with LIS. As we said earlier in Chapter Two, Dumas in his novel *The Count of Monte Cristo* described Monsieur Noirtier de Villefort (a character who had been "locked-in" for six years) as a "corpse with living eyes". As has been highlighted throughout this book, while a person with LIS will often have preserved vertical gaze and upper eyelid movement, this can be missed, certainly in the acute stages leading to misdiagnosis (see Chapter Four). This arguably leads to a number of ethical considerations in managing a person with LIS, including:

1 The delay in diagnosis and misdiagnosis.
2 The need to establish a form of reliable communication.
3 The issue of autonomy and decision making around refusal or acceptance of treatment.
4 The prevention of harm, in other words mitigating suffering.

1 Diagnosis

LIS can be mistakenly recognised as a vegetative state, minimally conscious state or akinetic mutism. It is often missed unless the treating medical professional is familiar with the signs and symptoms (Gallo and Fontanarosa 1989). Often the first person to recognise that the patient is attempting to communicate or attract attention is a family member (Leon-Carrion et al. 2002). This can be misunderstood by the healthcare staff as the family wanting to believe the patient is not in a disorder of consciousness. Given the delay of diagnosis and misdiagnosis there can be a significant time lapse between the initial brain insult and the diagnosis. In their survey of 44 LIS patients, Leon-Carrion et al. (2002) highlight that the time taken to diagnose was on average 2.5 months, with a number of patients not being diagnosed for over four years. Such delay not only causes significant stress and distress to the person in LIS but also to the family and friends, leading to impoverished quality of life and reduced psychological well-being. Wilson et al. (2011) highlight that delays in diagnosis can lead to insensitive bedside attitudes and the belief that the patient may be in a vegetative state. More importantly it can lead to delayed and/or incorrect rehabilitation and poor prognostic information. Inaccurate diagnosis is an ethical problem leading to biases in prognostic information and treatment strategies which in turn may lead to inappropriate decisions of withdrawal or withholding vital life-sustaining treatments (Laureys et al. 2005; Kuehlmeyer et al. 2011; Racine et al. 2010).

2 Communication

A person with LIS has intact consciousness and is relatively cognitively intact and, therefore, has the potential to communicate. However, in order for functional communication to be employed they remain dependent on others to facilitate communication. In order for the person to have autonomous decision making in everyday life and to be able to participate in their medical treatment, they are reliant on alternative communication aids and those around them to understand and translate their wishes accurately. It is therefore important that communication is established and is reliable.

In terms of medical intervention and treatment an individual, who has been deemed as competent to make medical decisions, has the right to make their own decisions around treatment without referring to the next of kin or treating team (Bruno et al. 2008). As research and anecdotal evidence has shown, patients with LIS are cognitively able (Leon-Carrion et al. 2002) and able to communicate their wishes (See Chapter 10). In the acute stage following brain insult, patients with LIS can be confronted with end-of-life decisions, and decisions around accepting or declining life-sustaining treatments such as artificial nutrition and artificial ventilation. These end-of-life decisions raise significant ethical issues. Their attitudes may be influenced by the treating physician and family members' opinions. These, in turn, will be influenced by how they perceive the patient's quality of life and, as mentioned in Chapter 10, most healthcare professionals, caregivers and relatives can often assume that quality of life of LIS patients is poor (Laureys et al. 2005).

Establishing communication using appropriate assessment, allowing sufficient time and being flexible in order to determine decision-making capacity in a patient with LIS is imperative. Innovative ways of communicating, including eye-tracking, fMRI technologies and brain computer interface systems, have been used in LIS. The proponents of such communication systems recognise that being able to communicate and to control the environment could influence not only their actual quality of life but also anticipated quality of life and, thus, their attitude towards end-of life decisions (Doble et al. 2003; Nijboer et al. 2006; Söderholm et al. 2001).

3 The issue of autonomy and decision making around refusal or acceptance of treatment

It is recognised the world over that patients have the *right* to make decisions with regard to medical treatments. Of course, they have to be assessed as competent and processes are in place to ensure appropriate decision making. In LIS this can be difficult and, in an attempt to support clinicians in managing conscious yet legally competent patients with profound paralysis (such as those with LIS), the American Academy of Neurology (AAN) published a position statement (Ethics and Humanities Subcommittee of the AAN; Bernat et al. 1993). They stated that these patients have the right to make healthcare decisions about themselves, including whether to accept or refuse life-sustaining therapy.

While the right of individuals to withdraw from treatment should not be questioned, establishing communication is imperative in enabling a patient with LIS to be autonomous and to be involved in decision making around refusal or acceptance of treatment. Without having a reliable method of communication, it can be difficult to determine whether or not the patient is making valid decisions of refusal or acceptance of treatment. This may lead to decisions being made on their behalf by families or treating teams which could be based on the assumption of poor quality of life. In a study conducted by Bruno et al. (2008) in which healthcare workers were surveyed around their perception of LIS, 66 per cent reported that they believed being locked-in would be worse than being in a vegetative or minimally conscious state. It has been argued that such perceptions could be significant, possibly encouraging reduced and less aggressive treatments or influencing the family to make inappropriate decisions (Doble et al. 2003). Furthermore, information on LIS may be ineffectively communicated and the available treatment options may not be provided (Ganzini and Block 2002).

There have been a number of case studies documented and investigated in the literature which have led to ethical debates regarding life-sustaining treatment and euthanasia (e.g. Jean-Dominique Bauby – see Bauby 1997; and Tony Nicklinson – see Miller 2012). There are studies that have shown that the majority of LIS patients do not wish to die and want life-sustaining treatments to be provided (e.g. Doble et al. 2003; Laureys et al. 2005). However, there are also some case reports and studies in which the patient desires death (e.g. Anderson et al. 2010). Such cases present healthcare professionals with an ethical dilemma, as euthanasia is illegal in nearly every country and is often viewed as an act of murder. This in turn leads to patients (e.g. in the case of Tony Nicklinson) having to fight the justice system in order to be "allowed" to die, which they see as their *right*, often without achieving a successful outcome of the fight.

4 The prevention of harm, in other words mitigating suffering

In all healthcare, there is a moral obligation to act for the benefit of others and prevent harm – the principle of beneficence. While the mitigation of suffering in LIS can often be seen as an end-of-life issue, it is a far bigger picture than that. As has been seen throughout this book people with LIS report *"a life worth living"* and therefore it is important that healthcare workers and policy makers understand long-term outcome of such patients. Patients with LIS need to be supported within a biopsychosocial model where their physical, psychological and social wellbeing is provided for, which in turn increases qualify of life and decreases suffering.

With appropriate medical care prognosis is good, with life expectancy being several decades. Many patients with LIS can return to their own homes. As has been previously discussed, LIS patients report a meaningful quality of life. Studies have shown that intensive and early rehabilitation can improve motor functions (Casanova et al. 2003). Advances in communication systems have enabled patients with LIS to "speak" and control their environments, something that previously was not possible (Nijboer et al. 2006).

Working with patients in LIS can give rise to many ethical challenges and healthcare professionals need to be prepared to deal with such challenges. Research suggests that the competence and cognitive abilities of LIS patients are too often underestimated. As a result they are not always involved in decision making around their own medical treatment options (Schnakers et al. 2008). Laureys et al. (2005, p. 348) argue that LIS patients need to be "exhaustively informed about their options to continue life (or not)".

It can be argued that in order to prevent harm, to mitigate suffering, that an understanding of the ability of patients with LIS to successfully adapt to their *new* life is imperative for all healthcare professionals. Without a comprehensive knowledge of LIS it is not possible to debate euthanasia and end-of-life issues (Schnakers et al. 2009). Ethical decisions need to be made in light of morbidity and survival literature and the medical and rehabilitation advances enabling patients with LIS to be able to live a fulfilled life. Research has provided evidence that life with LIS is worth living, something that Paul throughout this book attests to. However, in order to be able to do this, patients with LIS need communication and medical, emotional and social support from a treating team who understand what it is like to be locked-in from the perspective of the patient. Treating physicians need to challenge their own perceptions, beliefs and often distress in dealing with the ethical dilemmas that arise. By recognising the importance of determining decision-making capacity as early as possible following the brain insult, respecting patient autonomy and supporting patient choice and their right to live, LIS patients will be provided with the opportunity to regain a productive and meaningful life, albeit a new and different life.

12 Summary and conclusions

In this book we tell the story of Paul, who, at the age of 56 years, suffered a brain stem stroke which left him with Locked-In Syndrome (LIS). Despite intact cognitive abilities, he is unable to move his limbs, he has no voice, he is fed through a tube and requires regular ventilation. Even with these major physical limitations, Paul is fully engaged in life. He communicates through eye movements and has much to say; he is co-author of the current book and has another in press. His sense of humour is retained; he has good relationships with many people, including his wife, work colleagues, friends he has made through his love of music and singing, and people from the church. We hear from Paul's wife, Liz, who is a very important part of Paul's life. We also hear from some of his friends. They comment on his larger-than-life presence and how involved he was in so many shared activities.

Paul was an exceptionally good baritone singer and music was an essential part of his life. He remains interested in music, goes to concerts in a specially adapted wheelchair and has music therapy at the rehabilitation hospital where he was admitted soon after his stroke in 2012. In April 2017, Paul's friends put on a concert to celebrate Paul in which singers from the past 30 years of his singing career took part. We learnt how Paul became interested in music as a young child, how he joined a choir, of the singing parts he has played and some of his favourite musical memories.

To many people with full use of their limbs and their voice, the thought of being completely paralysed and unable to speak yet with their intellect intact seems too hard to bear. A large proportion of people when asked how they would feel if this happened to them say they would rather be dead. Yet most people who are locked-in do *not* feel this way. Paul is no exception. In addition to seeing his visitors regularly, he thinks about concerts; he sings in his head and can remember all the parts he has sung as well as everyone else's parts too. He has designed a big house for himself with a music room, a home cinema and a swimming pool. These "home truths" make us uneasy about living wills because what people think they will want after a major life-changing event changes once such an event has happened to them.

We address some of the other aspects of LIS, such as what it is, who is most at risk and can people recover from it. We also look at accounts of other people with LIS: those who have shown considerable recovery, those who have made some recovery and those who remain locked-in. We reflect on the length of time before LIS is diagnosed: for some people it takes years; for others, including Paul, it may be just a week or two before family members and carers realise there is understanding behind the paralysis and silence. Quality of life for people with LIS is another aspect we address. We look, too, at neuropsychological assessments of people with LIS and show that although there may be some subtle cognitive deficits, by and large, intellectual functioning is unimpaired. Sometimes, however, people may be locked-in *and* have additional cognitive problems. This may happen for example where there is cortical as well as brain stem damage such as may occur after a traumatic brain injury or hypoxic damage. If there are cognitive problems in addition to LIS, this can cause problems with diagnosis. We discuss two such cases where the neuropsychologists involved had difficulty coming to a decision as to whether patients had LIS or not. The assessments were confounded further by the fact that the two patients had problems controlling their eye movements.

This was not true of Paul. There is no doubt he has a good mind as he is well able to show it: he has learnt a few words in 26 languages and will often communicate in a foreign language through his blinking system. For example, he sometimes spells out "¿Cómo estás?" ("How are you?" in Spanish). As the person deciphering the blinking often predicts what word is likely to appear, foreign-language words can sometimes be confusing. This is one of the ways Paul teases. He is well able to tease and make jokes through his communication method.

The Mental Capacity Act (2005) says a person is deemed as not having capacity if they are unable to communicate. Paul, of course, is a good communicator, but one has to be prepared to go through the slow and sometimes laborious method of spelling out his words letter by letter, through his eye blinking. He is perfectly capable of making decisions about his life and his care. In other words, he has capacity. Notwithstanding this, the health authority paying for Paul's stay at the Raphael Hospital is reluctant to make home care possible through the provision of two full-time carers. Paul wishes to return home but also wishes to remain safe. This problem, too, is addressed in the book.

Our main message is to give a voice to a remarkable man who has LIS. His life is not pointless or worthless. He has much to tell us, much to contribute to the world, and we have much to learn from Paul. In many societies,

Summary and conclusions 83

people like Paul may well have been misdiagnosed or even died. Andrews (2005) and Wilson et al. (2016) report that we need to provide five conditions to promote optimal recovery for patients with profound brain damage. These are:

1   Provide the optimal environment.
2   Prevent and treat secondary complications.
3   Include in-treatment physiotherapy and the other "therapies", medical, psychological and technological.
4   Support the family.
5   Modify the environment – including regulating the amount of stimulation.

These authors were referring to people with a disorder of consciousness, but it can be argued that the same conditions need to be met for people with LIS too. It can be reasoned that these conditions *were*, by and large, met for Paul. He has not yet, though, at the time of writing (early 2018), returned home and this is largely because of financial reasons. This leaves one final goal that all of us working in rehabilitation should strive for – to persuade healthcare purchasers that rehabilitation and the best patient care makes clinical and economic sense. If we can save the lives of people with an insult to the brain, we owe it to them to make sure that the life we have saved is worth living.

References

Albrecht, G. L., & Devlieger, P. J. (1999). The disability paradox: high quality of life against all odds. *Social Science & Medicine, 48*(8), 977–988.
Allain, P., Joseph, P. A., Isambert, J. L., Le Gall, D., & Emile, J. (1998). Cognitive functions in chronic locked-in syndrome: a report of two cases. *Cortex, 34*, 629–634.
Allatt, K., & Stokes, A. (2011) *Running Free: Breaking Out from Locked-In Syndrome*. Cardiff, UK: Accent Press Ltd.
Al-Raweshidy, Y. H., Sinha, D. M., Coward, L. J., Guyler, P. C., & O'Brien, A. (2011). Locked in and out: a case of emerging basilar artery obstruction secondary to vertebral artery dissection thrombolysed with intravenous rt-PA. *BMJ Case Reports*. doi:10.1136/bcr.12.2010.3584.
American Congress of Rehabilitation Medicine. (1995). Recommendations for use of uniform nomenclature pertinent to patients with severe alterations of consciousness. *Archives of Physical Medicine and Rehabilitation, 76*, 205–209.
American Speech-Language-Hearing Association. (n.d.) Frequently Asked Questions (FAQ) about tracheotomy and swallowing. Retrieved from http://www.asha.org/SLP/clinical/Frequently-Asked-Questions-on-Tracheotomy-and-Swallowing/
Anderson, C., Dillon, C., & Burns, R. (1993). Life-sustaining treatment and locked-in syndrome. *Lancet, 342*, 867–868.
Anderson, J. F. I., Augoustakis, L. V., Holmes, R. J., & Chambers, B. R. (2010). End-of-life decision-making in individuals with Locked-in syndrome in the acute period after brainstem stroke. *Internal Medicine Journal, 40*(1), 61–65.
Andrews, K. (2005). Rehabilitation practice following profound brain damage. *Neuropsychological Rehabilitation, 15*, 461–472.
Annen, J., Laureys, S., & Gosseries, O. (2017). People with Disorders of Consciousness. In Wilson, B. A., Winegardner, J., van Heugten, C., & Ownsworth, T. (eds) *Neuropsycholgical Rehabilitation: An International Handbook*. London: Routledge, pp. 124–135.
Baddeley A. D, Emslie, H., & Nimmo-Smith, I. (1993). The Spot-the-Word test: a robust estimate of verbal intelligence based on lexical decision. *The British Journal of Clinical Psychology, 32*, 55–65.
Baddeley, A. D., Nimmo-Smith, I., & Emslie, H. (1994). *Doors and People*. Bury St Edmunds, UK: Thames Valley Test Company.

Bauby, J.-D. (1997). *The Diving Bell and the Butterfly* (original title: *Le scaphandre et le papillon*, Robert Laffont, Paris), New York. KNOPF.
Bauer, G., Gerstenbrand, F., & Rumpl, E. (1979). Varieties of the locked-in syndrome. *Journal of Neurology*, *221*, 77–91.
Beaudoin, N., & De Serres, L. (2010). Locked-In Syndrome. In Stone, J. H., & Blouin, M. (eds) *International Encyclopedia of Rehabilitation*. Retrieved from http://cirrie.buffalo.edu/encyclopedia/en/article/303/
Beaumont, J. G., Marjoribanks, J., Flury, S., & Lintern, T. (2002). *Putney Auditory Comprehension Screening Test* (PACST) London: Harcourt Assessment.
Bernat, J. L., Cranford, R. E., Kittredge, F. I., & Rosenberg, R. N. (1993). Competent patients with advanced states of permanent paralysis have the right to forgo life-sustaining therapy. *Neurology*, *43*(1), 224–224.
Bishop, D. (2003). *The Test for Reception of Grammar*, 2nd edition. London: Pearson Assessment.
Bruno, M., Bernheim, J. L., Schnakers, C., & Laureys, S. (2008a). Locked-in: don't judge a book by its cover. *Journal of Neurology, Neurosurgery & Psychiatry*, *79*(1), 2–2.
Bruno, M. A., Pellas, F., Schnakers, C., Van Eeckhout, P., Bernheim, J., Pantke, K. H., Damas, F., Faymonville, M. E., Moonen, G., Goldman, S., & Laureys, S. (2008b). Blink and you live: the locked-in syndrome. *Revue Neurologique (Paris)*, *164*(4), 322–35.
Bruno, M. A., Bernheim, J. L., Ledoux, D., Pellas, F., Demertzi, A., & Laureys, S. (2011). A survey on self-assessed well-being in a cohort of chronic locked-in syndrome patients: happy majority, miserable minority. *BMJ Open*, *1*(1), e000039.
Cappa, S. F., & Vignolo, L. A. (1982). Locked-in syndrome for 12 years with preserved intelligence. *Annals of Neurology*, *11*(5), 545.
Cappa, S. F., Pirovano, C., & Vignolo, L. A. (1985). Chronic 'locked-in' syndrome: psychological study of a case. *European Neurology*, *24*(2), 107–111.
Carrington, S., & Birns, J. (2012). Establishing capacity in a patient with incomplete locked-in syndrome. *Progress in Neurology and Psychiatry*, *16*(6), 18–20.
Casanova, E., Lazzari, R. E., Lotta, S., & Mazzucchi, A. (2003). Locked-in Syndrome: improvement in the prognosis after an early intensive multidisciplinary rehabilitation. *Archives of Physical Medicine and Rehabilitation*, *84*, 862–7.
Chisholm, N., & Gillett, G. (2005). The patient's journey: living with locked-in syndrome. *British Medical Journal*, *331*, 94–97.
Coghlan, P. (2013). *In the Blink of an Eye*. Retrieved from www.petercoghlan.com
Darolles, M. (1875). Ramolissement de la protubérance: thrombose du tronc basilaire. *Le Progrès Médicate*, *3*, 629–639.
Davies, A., Davies, B., & Davies, E. (2015). *Pressed but Not Crushed*. Welwyn Garden City, UK: Malcolm Down Publishing Ltd.
Delis, D. C., Kramer, J. H., Kaplan, E., & Ober, B. A. (1987). *California Verbal Learning Test: Adult Version*. San Antonio, TX: The Psychological Corporation.
Doble, J. E., Haig, A. J., Anderson, C., & Katz, R. (2003). Impairment, activity, participation, life satisfaction, and survival in persons with locked-in syndrome for over a decade: follow-up on a previously reported cohort. *The Journal of Head Trauma Rehabilitation*, *18*, 435–444.

References

Duffy, J. R. (2000) Motor Speech Disorders: Clues to Neurologic Diagnosis. In Adler, C. H., & Ahlskog, J. E. (eds) *Parkinson's Disease and Movement Disorders*. Current Clinical Practice Series. Totowa, NJ: Humana Press, pp. 35–53.

Dumas, A. (1844). *The Count of Monte Cristo*. Paris: Petion.

Gallo, U. E., & Fontanarosa, P. B. (1989). Locked-in syndrome: report of a case. *The American Journal of Emergency Medicine*, 7(6), 581–583.

Ganzini, L., & Block, S. (2002). Physician-assisted death – a last resort? *New England Journal of Medicine*, 346, 1663–1665.

Garrard, P., Bradshaw, D., Jager, H. R., Thompson, A. J., Losseff, N., & Playford, D. (2002). Cognitive dysfunction after isolated brain stem insult: an underdiagnosed cause of long-term morbidity. *Journal of Neurology, Neurosurgy, and Psychiatry*, 73, 191–194.

Ghorbel, S. (unpublished). Statut fonctionnel et qualité de vie chez le locked-in syndrome a domicile. In *DEA Motricité Humaine et Handicap, Laboratory of Biostatistics, Epidemiology and Clinical Research*. Dissertation in Medicine. Université Jean Monnet Saint- Étienne, Montpellier, France.

Goode, D. (ed.). (1994). *Quality of Life for Persons with Disabilities: International Perspectives and Issues*. Cambridge, MA: Brookline.

Hocker, S., Eelco, F. M., & Wijdicks, M. D. (2015). Recovery from Locked-in Syndrome. *JAMA Neurology*, 72, 832–833.

Huskisson, E. C. (1974). Measurement of pain. *Lancet*, 2(7889), 1127–1131.

Katz, R. T., Haig, A. J., Clark, B. B., & DiPaola, R. J. (1992). Long-term survival, prognosis, and life-care planning for 29 patients with chronic locked-in syndrome. *Archives of Physical Medicine and Rehabilitation*, 73, 403–408.

Kopelman, M. D., Wilson, B. A., & Baddeley, A. D. (1990). *The Autobiographical Memory Interview*. Bury St Edmunds, UK: Thames Valley Test Company.

Kübler, A., Winter, S., Ludolph, A. C., Hautzinger, M., & Birbaumer, N. (2005). Severity of depressive symptoms and quality of life in patients with amyotrophic lateral sclerosis. *Neurorehabilitation and neural Repair*, 19(3), 182–193.

Kuehlmeyer, K., Racine, E., Palmour, N., Hoster, E., Borasio, G. D., & Jox, R. J. (2012). Diagnostic and ethical challenges in disorders of consciousness and locked-in syndrome: a survey of German neurologists. *Journal of Neurology*, 259(10), 2076–2089.

Laureys, S., Pellas, F., Van Eeckhout, P., Ghorbel, S., Schnakers, C., Perrin, F., Berre, F., Faymonville, M.-E., Pantke, K.-H., Damas, F., Lamy, M., Moonen, G., & Goldman, S. (2005). The locked-in syndrome: what is it like to be conscious but paralyzed and voiceless? In S. Laureys (ed.) *Progress in Brain Research Vol 150*. Amsterdam: Elsevier, pp. 495–451

Laureys, S., Perrin, F., & Bredart, S. (2007). Self-consciousness in non-communicative patients. *Consciousness and Cognition*, 16, 722–741.

Leon-Carrion, J., van Eeckhout, P., Dominguez-Morales, M. D. R., & Perez-Santamaria, F. J. (2002). The locked-in syndrome: a syndrome looking for a therapy. *Brain Injury*, 16, 571–582.

Leplege, A., Ecosse, E., Verdier, A., & Perneger, T. V. (1998). The French SF-36 Health Survey: translation, cultural adaptation and preliminary psychometric evaluation. *Journal of Clinical Epidemiology*, 51, 1013–1023.

Lulé, D., Zickler, C., Häcker, S., Bruno, M. A., Demertzi, A., Pellas, F., ... & Kübler, A. (2009). Life can be worth living in locked-in syndrome. *Progress in Brain Research*, *177*, 339–351.

Maiser, S., Kabir A., Sabsevitz D., & Peltier, W. (2016). Locked-in syndrome: case report and discussion of decisional capacity. *Journal of Pain Symptom Management*, *51*(4), 789–793.

Marjerus, S., Van Der Linden, M., & Shiel, A. (2000). The Wessex Head Injury Matrix and the Glasgow/Glasgow-Liege coma scale: a validation and comparison study. *Neuropsychological Rehabilitation*, *10*, 167–184.

Marsh, R., & Hudson, J. (2014). *One Man's Miraculous Escape from the Terrifying Confines of Locked-In Syndrome*. London: Piatkus.

McGee, H. M., O'Boyle, C. A., Hickey, A., O'Malley, K., & Joyce, C. R. B. (1991). Assessing the quality of life of the individual: the SEIQoL with a healthy and a gastroenterology unit population. *Psychological Medicine*, *21*(3), 749–759.

Mental Capacity Act. (2005). Department of Health: London, Her Majesty's Stationery Office.

Miller, D. (2012, 19 June). My life is miserable, demeaning and undignified says locked-in syndrome sufferer as he asks High Court judges to give him the right to die. Retrieved 21 January 2018 from *Mail Online* website, http://www.dailymail.co.uk/news/article-2161494/Tony-Nicklinson-euthanasia-My-life-miserable-undignified-says-locked-syndrome-sufferer.html

Moons, P., Budts, W., & De Geest, S. (2006). Critique on the conceptualization of quality of life: a review and evaluation of different conceptual approaches. *International Journal of Nursing Studies*, *43*, 891–901.

Murphy, L. (in press). Cognitive and psychological profiles of people emerging from disorders of consciousness: towards an assessment framework. *Neuropsychological Rehabilitation*.

Murphy, M. J., Brenton, D. W., Aschenbrener, C. A., & Van Gilder, J. C. (1979). Locked-in syndrome caused by a solitary pontine abscess. *Journal of Neurology, Neurosurgery, and Psychiatry*, *42*, 1062–1065. doi:10.1136/jnnp.42.11.1062.

Murrell, R. (1999). Quality of life and neurological illness: a review of the literature. *Neuropsychology Review*, *9*(4), 209–229.

National Organization for Rare Disorders (NORD) (2016).

Nelson, H. E. (1976). A modified card sorting test sensitive to frontal lobe defects. *Cortex; a Journal Devoted to the Study of the Nervous System and Behavior*, *12*(4), 313–324.

New, P. W., & Thomas, S. J. (2005). Cognitive impairments in the locked-in syndrome: a case report. *Archives of Physical Medicine and Rehabilitation*, *86*, 338–343.

Nijboer, F., Matuz, T., Kübler, A., & Birbaumer, N. (2006, September). Ethical, psychological and social implications of brain-computer interface application in paralyzed patients. *AAI Workshop*.

O'Reilly, A. (2014). *Out of the Darkness*. Bloomington, IN: Archway Publishing.

Patterson, J. R., & Grabois, M. (1986). Locked-in syndrome: a review of 139 cases. *Stroke*, *17*, 758–764.

Pierrot-Deseilligny, C., Milea, D., & Muri, R. M. (2004). Eye movement control by the cerebral cortex. *Current Opinion in Neurology*, *17*, 17–25.

Pink, K. (2010). I lay paralysed and unable to speak for 18 months. *Daily Mail*, 5 August.
Pistorius, M., & Davies, M. L. (2011). *Ghost Boy*. London: Simon and Schuster.
Plum, F., & Posner, J. B. (1966). *The Diagnosis of Stupor and Coma*. Philadelphia, PA: FA Davis.
Plum, F. & Posner, J. B. (1983). *The Diagnosis of Stupor and Coma*. Philadelphia, PA: FA Davis.
Racine, E., Rodrigue, C., Bernat, J. L., Riopelle, R., & Shemie, S. D. (2010). Observations on the ethical and social aspects of disorders of consciousness. *Canadian Journal of Neurological Sciences*, *37*(6), 758–768.
Ratcliff, G. (1979). Spatial thought, mental rotation and the right cerebral hemisphere. *Neuropsychologia*, *17*(1), 49–54.
Raven, J. C. (1982). *Revised Manual for Raven's Progressive Matrices*. Windsor, Berkshire: NFER-Nelson.
Rousseaux, M., Castelnot, E., Rigaux, P., Kozlowski, O., & Danzé, F. (2009). Evidence of persisting cognitive impairment in a case series of patients with locked-in syndrome. *Journal of Neurology, Neurosurgery, and Psychiatry*, *80*(2), 166–170.
Rousseau, M. C., Pietra, S., Blaya, J., & Catala, A. (2011). Quality of life of ALS and LIS patients with and without invasive mechanical ventilation. *Journal of Neurology*, *258*(10), 1801–1804.
Rousseau, M. C., Pietra, S., Nadji, M., & Billette de Villemeur, T. (2013). Evaluation of quality of life in complete locked-in syndrome patients. *Journal of Palliative Medicine*, *16*(11), 1455–1458.
Schnakers, C., Majerus, S., Van Eeckhout, P., Peigneux, P., & Laureys, S. (2004). Neuropsychological testing in the locked-in syndrome: preliminary results from a feasibility study. *Critical Care*, *8*(Suppl 1), 314.
Schnakers, C., Majerus, S., Goldman, S., Boly, M., Van Eeckhout, P., Gay, S., Pellas, F., Bartsch, V., Peigneux, P., Moonen, G., & Laureys, S. (2008). Cognitive function in the locked-in syndrome. *Journal of Neurology*, *255*, 323–330.
Schnakers, C., Vanhaudenhuyse, A., Giacino, J., Ventura, M., Boly, M., Majerus, S., & Laureys, S. (2009). Diagnostic accuracy of the vegetative and minimally conscious state: clinical consensus versus standardized neurobehavioral assessment. *BMC Neurology*, *9*(1), 35.
Seligman, M. (2011). *Flourish*. London: Nicholas Brearley Publishing.
Shallice, T., & Burgess, P. W. (1997). *The Hayling and Brixton Tests*. Bury St Edmunds, UK: Thames Valley Test Company.
Sharma, P., Busby, M., Chapple, L., Matthews, R., & Chapple, I. (2016). The relationship between general health and lifestyle factors and oral health outcomes *British Dental Journal*, *221*, 65–69.
Shiel, A., Wilson, B. A., McLellan, L., Horn, S., & Watson, M. (2000). *The Wessex Head Injury Matrix (WHIM)*. Bury St Edmunds, UK: Thames Valley Test Company.
Smart, C. M., Giacino, J. T, Cullen, T., Rodriguez Moreno, D., Hirsch, J., Schiff, N. D., & Gizzi, M. (2008). A case of locked-in syndrome complicated by central deafness. *Nature Clinical Practice Neurology*, *4*, 448–453.
Smith, E., & Delargy, M. (2005). Clinical review: locked-in syndrome. *British Medical Journal*, *330*, 406–409.

Söderholm, S., Meinander, M., & Alaranta, H. (2001). Augmentative and alternative communication methods in locked-in syndrome. *Journal of Rehabilitation Medicine, 33*(5), 235–239.

Tavalaro, J., & Tayson, R. (1997). *Look Up for Yes*. New York: Ko-dansha America Inc.

Trojano, L., Moretta, P., Estraneo, A., & Santoro, L. (2010). Neuropsychologic assessment and cognitive rehabilitation in a patient with locked-in syndrome and left neglect. *Archives of Physical Medicine and Rehabilitation, 91*(3), 498–502.

Vigand, P., & Vigand, S. (2000). Only the Eyes Say Yes (original title: *Putain de silence*). New York: Arcade Publishing.

Ware, J. E., Snow, K. K., & Kosinski, M. (1993). *SF-36 Health Survey Manual and Interpretation Guide*. Boston, MA: The Health Institute, New England Medical Center.

Ware, J E., Kosinski, M., & Dewey, J. E. (2000). *How to Score Version 2 of the SF-36*. Lincoln, RI: Quality Metric Incorporated.

Warrington, E. K. (1984). *Recognition Memory Test*. Windsor, UK: NFER-Nelson Windsor.

Warrington, E. K., & McKenna, P. (1980). *The Graded Naming Test*. Cambridge: Cambridge Cognition.

Warrington, E. K., & James, M. (1991). *The Visual Object and Space Perception Battery*. Bury St Edmunds, UK: Thames Valley Test Company.

Wechsler, D. (2008). *Wechsler Adult Intelligence Scale-IV*. San Antonio, TX: Psychological Corporation.

Wilson, B. A., Greenfield, E., Clare, L., Baddeley, A. D., Cockburn, J., Watson, P., Tate, R., Sopena, S., & Nannery, R. (2008). *The Rivermead Behavioural Memory Test – 3*. London: Pearson Assessment.

Wilson, B. A., Hinchcliffe, A., Okines, T., Florschutz, G., & Fish, J. (2011). A case study of Locked-In Syndrome: psychological and personal perspectives. *Brain Injury, 25*, 526–538.

Wilson, B. A., & Okines, T. (2014). Tracey's Story: Quality of life with Locked-In Syndrome. In Wilson, B. A., Winegardner, J., & Ashworth, F. (eds) *Life after Brain Injury: Survivors' Stories*. Hove, UK: Psychology Press, pp. 75–83.

Wilson, B. A., Dhamapurkar, S., & Rose, A. (2016). *Surviving Brain Injury after Assault: Gary's Story*. Hove, UK: Psychology Press.

Zigmond, A. S., & Snaith, R. P. (1983). The Hospital Anxiety and Depression Scale. *Acta Psychiatrica Scandinavica, 67*(6), 361–370.

Zola, E. (1867). *Thérèse Raquin*. Paris: Delacroix.

Appendices

Appendix One

TRANSFER PROTOCOL

Name of patient: Paul Allen   **DOB:** 13/01/1956

Room no.: Tobias House No. 1

Type of transfer: Hoist transfer

Assistance required: Two persons

Equipment required: Skyframe ceiling hoist; Silvalea Deluxe, Medium sling

Protocol:

1. Check the hoist to make sure it is working, i.e. battery charged and remote functional, appropriate hoist and sling is used and ensure the surface to which the patient is transferred is ready.
2. Explain the procedure to Paul and gain his consent.
3. Check to ensure that the sling is placed properly on Paul.
4. Hook the sling to the hoist. (Select the position of hooks depending on the position Paul is going for, i.e. select the second hook on upper (head side) part of sling if he is going to lie down.) The sling has two hooks on upper part (head side) and one hook in the lower part (leg side).
5. Inform Paul before the remote control switch is pressed.
6. If possible, move the empty surface to the hoist.
7. Once Paul is properly over the transferring surface, warn him and lower the hoist. When transferring to wheelchair, make sure it is in tilt before you transfer him onto it to obtain optimal sitting posture.
8. Unhook the sling after making sure Paul is safe and properly positioned.

NB: Transfer should be carried out by trained staff at all times. Ensure that the transfer is done by two staff. The NIPPY ventilator remains at the back of the wheelchair or his side table, so ensure the tubing is handled carefully. Staff should ensure that the respirator tube is attached all the time and is properly functioning according to recommended readings as well as the tracheostomy tube is not being dragged to one side and remains in the middle. Reattach the tube immediately in the event of detachment from connector.

Appendix Two

PRINCIPLES FOR SEATED POSITIONING

1. Ensure that Paul's body is aligned at all times, i.e. head, neck, spine, pelvis and lower limbs are maintained in straight alignment. Ensure that his pelvis is placed at the back of the seat against the backrest, maintaining an anterior pelvic tilt at all times. Look and check there are no gaps between Paul's back and the backrest. If necessary, reposition Paul after he is transferred into the chair.
2. Ensure there is one pillow to support. Arms and elbow should be supported on arm rest: one pillow to be placed on lap to support hands optimally.
3. Ensure Paul's knees are in a straight line with his hips – therefore the knees are not rubbing together or flopped to the side.
4. Ensure that the seatbelt is always securely fastened.
5. Shoes must be worn at all times and feet are to be placed correctly on footrests.
6. Paul prefers to sit reclined backwards. Recline should be between 60°–75°. Always ask Paul is he requires further adjusting.
7. Always ask Paul whether he is overall comfortable after positioning. This is very important.

Index

accident and emergency (A & E) 34, 43
activities of daily living (ADLs)
  45, 52
Albrecht, G. L. 70
Allain, P. 10, 13
Allatt, K. 2, 6–7, 10
Al-Raweshidy, Y. H. 3
American Academy of Neurology
  (AAN) 78
American Congress of Rehabilitation
  Medicine 1, 21, 27
American Speech-Language-Hearing
  Association (AHSA) 47
Anderson, C. x
Anderson, J. F. I. 79
Andrews, K. 83
Annen, J. 21
Autobiographical Memory Interview
  17, 19

Baddeley, A. D. 16, **19**
basilar artery 1–3, 11, 43; occlusion 1,
  11, 14, 18, 44; thrombosis ix, 9
Bauby, J.-D. xi, 3, 5, 78
Bauer, G. 1, 26
Beaudoin, N. x, 2
Beaumont, J. G. 26
Bernat, J. L. 78
Bishop, D. **19**
blinking 1, 3, 5–8, 13, 21–27, 38–39,
  42, 58, 67, 73, 82
board *see also* communication: letter 6,
  9, 15; spelling 7
brain damage 1; profound 83
brain injury xii, 2, 21, 25; traumatic
  (TBI), 22, 82

Brixton Spatial Anticipation Test 15,
  17, 20
Bruno, M. A. 2, 69, 77–78

California Verbal Learning Test 15–16, 19
Cappa, S. F. 13
Carrington, S. 74
Casanova, E. 2–3, 79
case studies: M.A. 21–24, 26–27;
  U.P. 24–27
Chisholm, N. 2, 8, 10
Coghlan, P. 2, 6–7
cognitive: abilities x, 1, 21, 27, 73–74,
  79, 81; assessment xii, 15, 17, 53;
  deficits 13–15, 18, 26, 82; domain 14;
  function 13–15; problem 24, 26–27, 82
Cognitive Assessment by Visual
  Election (CAVE) 26
coma xii, 6, 9, 11, 21–22, 34, 36–37
comatose xii, 6–8, 10
communication: aid 39, 69, 73, 75, 77;
  augmented 6; board 9, 13, 15, 39;
  device 6, 13, 15; verbal 3
computer x, xii, 3, 6, 30–31, 49, 62, 67,
  77; game 7, 9; programmer 30
continuing health care 65–66
cranial nerve 1, 44

Darolles, M. 5
Davies, A. 2–3, 6–7
Delis, D. C. 16, **19**
Doble, J. E. x, 2, 69, 78
Doors and People Test 13, 16, 18
Duffy, J. R. 27
Dumas, A. 5, 76
dysphagia 49–50

Index 93

emotional 18, 39, 61, 70–71, **71**; problems 18, 70–71; support 55–56, 80; well-being 17, 53, 55–56, 70–71, **71**
eye movements x–xi, 1, 13, 15, 21, 23–24, 27, 81–82 *see also* blinking; lateral 1, 21; vertical 1, 15, 21

French Locked-in Syndrome Society 9
functioning *see also* cognitive, neuropsychological: executive 13–15, 17–18, **20**, 53; physical 70, **71**; premorbid 15, 18, **19**, 53; role **71**; social 70, **71**; visuo-spatial 15, **20**

Gallo, U. E. 76
Ganzini, L. 69, 78
Garrard, P. 8, 10, 14, 16
Ghorbel, S. 69
Glasgow Coma Scale 43
Goode, D. 68

haemorrhage 5, 24; pontine 1–2, 22
healthcare 74, 78–79, 83; professionals 72, 74, 77, 79; teams x; workers 76, 78–79
Hocker, S. 3
Hospital Anxiety and Depression Scale 17
Huskisson, E. C. 17

intensive: care unit (ICU) xii, 34, 36, 58; treatment unit (ITU) 43

Katz, R. T. 3
Kopelman, M. D. 17, **19**
Kübler, A. 69
Kuehlmeyer, K. 77

language 5, 15, 18, **19**, 22, 25–26, 49, 53, 55, 66, 73, 82 *see also* speech and language therapy
Laureys, S. x, 5, 69, 77–79
Leon-Carrion, J. 14, 21, 76–77
Leplege, A. 70–71
locked in syndrome (LIS): classical 1; partial 1, 26–27; total 1, 3, 26
Lulé, D. 69

McGee, H. M. 69
Maiser, S. 74
Manikin Test 16, 18, 20
Marjerus, S. 22
Marsh, R. 2, 6, 8
matrix reasoning 16, 18, 20
memory 8, 13–18, **19**, 27, 53; verbal 14, 16–17; visual 14, 16, 53
mental capacity 42, 73–74
Mental Capacity Act 72–74, 82
Miller, D. 78
Modified Card Sorting Test 15, 20
Moons, P. 69
Murphy, L. 26
Murphy, M. J. 79
Murrell, R. 69
muscles: eye 23–24, 26; facial 47; neck 17; tone 47–48; voluntary 1

National Organization for Rare Disorders (NORD) 1–2
Nelson, H. E. 15, **20**
Neuro Functional Reorganisational Therapy (NFRT) 50
neuropsychological: assessment 13–15, 22, 24, 74, 82; functioning 15; test 13, 15, **19**, 21
New, P. W. 10, 14, 16
Nicklinson, T. 78–79
Nijboer, F. 78–79
Nippy machine (ventilator) 44, 46–47, 55, 91
nystagmus 25, 44

Okines, T. (Tracey) 3, 7, 9–10, 15–18, **19–20**, 21, 53, 69
ophthalmoplegia 24, 26–27
O'Reilly, A. 3, 6–7

paralysis xii, 1, 8, 10, 18, 22, 26, 44, 51, 71, 78, 82
passive range of movement (PROM) 47–48
Patterson, J. R. 1
perception 14, 16–17, 68, 78, 80 *see also* Visual Object and Space Perception Battery; visual 15–16, 25
percutaneous endoscopic gastrostomy (PEG) 44–45, 47, 49, 51

picture completion 16, 18, 20, 53
Pierrot-Deseilligny, C. 27
Pink, K. 2, 8
Pistorius, M. 3, 6
Plum, F. 1
pneumonia 2, 6–7, 38
power of attorney (POA) 37
Princess Royal Hospital (PRUH) 38–40
Putney Auditory Comprehension Screening Test (PACST) 26

quadriplegia 1, 21, 44
quality of life (QOL) x, xii, 8, 17–18, 51, 53, 56, 68–71, 75, 77–79, 82

Racine, E. 77
Raphael Hospital 34, 38–39, 42, 51, 53, 57–59, 62, 65–66, 71, 75, 82; Tobias House 34
Ratcliff, G. 16, **20**
Raven, J. C. 16, **20**
Ravens Matrices 16, 18, **20**, 53

reasoning 8, 15–16, 18, **20**, 53
recovery xii, 2–4, 7–8, 14, 82–83
rehabilitation iii, xii, 7, 18, 24, 34, 42, 74–75, 77, 79, 81, 83; neuro- iii, 3, 42
Rivermead Behavioural Memory Test-3 (RBMT) 16, 18, 19
Rousseau, M. C. 69
Rousseaux, M. 14

scan 11, 15–16, 18, 25, 43, 51; CT (computerised tomography) 9, 11, 22, 34–37, 43; MRI (magnetic resonance imaging) 9, 37, 77
Schnakers, C. 2, 13–14, 18, 79
Seligman, M. 75
Shallice, T. 15, **20**
Sharma, P. 2
Shiel, A. 22
Short Form-36 Health Survey (SF-36) 17, 70, 71
Smart, C. M. 1, 13, 15
Smith, E. x, 1, 13–16, 73
Söderholm, S. 78
speech and language therapy (SALT) xii, 6, 15, 24, 26, 42, 49–52

stroke ix–xi, 1–3, 6–8, 10–11, 14–15, 21–22, 28, 31, 34–41, 44, 58–59, 61, 63, 65, 71, 81; brain stem 2, 5, 7–8, 81
survival/survivor x–xi, 2–3, 5, 7, 9, 11, 66, 79, 85
swallowing 3, 7, 44, 47, 49–51

Tavalaro, J. 3, 5–6, 21
therapy *see also* speech and language therapy: art 42, 55–56; music xii, 42, 56–57, 67, 81; occupational (OT) xii, 6, 39, 42, 52; physio- xii, 22, 42, 47–52, 66, 83
THERA-Trainer 47–49
tracheostomy 3, 11, 24, 40, 44, 46, 50, 66, 74, 91
trauma 2, 14, 22, 33 *see also* brain injury
Trojano, L. 13, 15

verbal 14, 16, 24, 73–74 *see also* communication, memory
Vigand, P. 3, 6
visual analogue scale (VAS) 17
Visual Object and Space Perception Battery (VOSP) 16, 18
voice 1, 5–6, 21, 23, 31, 37, 40, 47, 59, 73–74, 81–82

Ware, J. E. 17, 70
Warrington, E. K. 16–17, **19–20**
Warrington's Recognition Memory Test 16–17
Wechsler, D. 16, 20
Wechsler Adult Intelligence Scale (WAIS) 16, 18, 20
Wessex Head Injury Matrix (WHIM) 22, 24
wheelchair 2–3, 9, 48, 52, 54, 64, 81, 90–91
Wilson, B. A. xii, 3, 7, 9, 12–13, 15–16, **19**, 42, 57, 67, 69, 77, 83
Wisconsin Card Sorting Test 13, 17
World Health Organisation (WHO) 68

Zigmond, A. S. 17
Zola, E. 5